DIABETES
SUCKS
AND YOU CAN HANDLE IT

YOUR GUIDE to MANAGING the
EMOTIONAL CHALLENGES of T1D

MARK HEYMAN
PHD CDCES

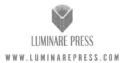

LUMINARE PRESS
WWW.LUMINAREPRESS.COM

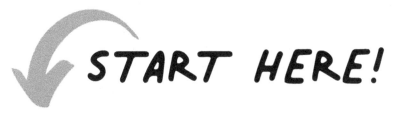

START HERE!

Want a roadmap to help you get the most out of this book?

Download this free guide!

In this guide, I'll help you identify:

1.

Your biggest challenge with T1D
It may not be what you think

2.

What you want to do in your life with T1D
You'll dream big

3.

A clear path to get you there
Small steps lead to big progress

Go to www.thediabetespsychologist.com/ roadmap or scan the code below to download this guide now!

SCAN ME

Printed in the United States of America

Luminare Press
442 Charnelton St.
Eugene, OR 97401
www.luminarepress.com

LCCN: 2022901626
ISBN: 978-1-64388-873-6

To Gayle and Hannah

TABLE OF CONTENTS

INTRODUCTION

LET'S BE COMPLETELY honest with each other.

Life with type 1 diabetes (T1D) is HARD.

Never let anyone tell you it isn't.

I know how challenging it can be to deal with T1D every single day. I'm certainly never going to tell you that life with T1D is easy. I'm also never going to tell you that what you are feeling isn't real or that you shouldn't let yourself feel burned out, worried, overwhelmed, anxious, or whatever other emotions T1D brings up.

I know you are doing the best you can with the resources you have. You probably have tried everything you can think of to make T1D less stressful. Some of these strategies may have helped you in the short term, but they haven't given you the lasting relief you're hoping to find.

I have some good news for you!

Things can get better. Life with T1D doesn't have to be such a big struggle. This book is going to show you how.

About Dr. Mark

Before we go any further, let me introduce myself.

My name is Dr. Mark Heyman—most people call me Dr. Mark. I am a clinical psychologist, and I specialize in helping people navigate the emotional challenges of living with T1D. I understand T1D not only professionally but also personally—I've been living with T1D for over 20 years.

I know exactly what life with T1D is like because I live it every day. I also have more than ten years of experience helping people keep the emotional burden from getting in their way. I know you are struggling right now, and I also know a thing or two about how to help you navigate these struggles.

My Diabetes Story

I was diagnosed with type 1 diabetes on June 1, 1999. It was the end of my junior year of college, and I was just finishing an intense quarter. In addition to taking a full load of classes, I also was campaigning for student government (I lost) and was getting ready to spend the summer in Paris.

I had dreamed of traveling to France since I was in high school and finally had the opportunity. I got an internship at the U.S. Embassy in Paris. I would be working during the day and exploring Paris at night and on the weekends. I couldn't wait—the summer couldn't arrive fast enough!

And then I got sick.

At first, I had an unquenchable thirst and found myself constantly in the bathroom. Then, I started losing weight and was having trouble concentrating. Every day I told myself this was temporary and that the next day would be better.

It wasn't.

Every day I felt worse. It was obvious there was something wrong with me and that I needed help. But I was terrified. If I was as sick as I felt, that meant my summer in Paris would be canceled, and I wasn't ready to accept this possibility.

That first day of June was my breaking point. I remember walking to class but couldn't make it up the hill. I knew I needed help, so I dragged myself over to student health. After sitting in the waiting room for what felt like forever—with frequent trips to the drinking fountain and the restroom—I finally was called to the exam room. When the doctor walked in, I told him my symptoms. Without missing a beat, he walked out of the room and returned with a blood glucose meter. He pricked my finger and after a minute-long wait...

The meter said HI—my blood sugar was over 600mg/dl.

The rest of that day was a blur. The student health center called an ambulance, and they rushed me to the emergency room. After several hours, the doctor came in and told me I had T1D, and then they sent me home with an appointment to see an endocrinologist the next day.

The entire time I was at the hospital, my mind was racing as I tried to wrap my head around what this news meant for my summer plans. Being diagnosed with T1D was terrible news on its own, but the thought of having to cancel my trip to France was devastating.

The following morning, I walked into my new endocrinologist's office. She spent several hours giving me a crash course in T1D. I was overwhelmed and didn't take in a word she said until the end of our appointment when she asked if I had any questions. That's when my heart started racing.

I finally had the chance to make my case.

I was nervous, but I started telling the doctor about my plans to go to Paris for the summer. Just as I started to ask her whether it might be possible to salvage the trip, she stopped me in the middle of my pity party and asked why I would have to cancel.

The doctor had no doubt I could go to Paris that summer. She told me T1D is not easy, but she was confident I could handle it.

Those words have been my motto ever since.

Eighteen days after I was diagnosed with T1D, I boarded a plane and flew to Paris. I had the time of my life that summer in France. I can't say it was easy, but I did it. All these years later, I remember that trip well, and very few of those memories have anything to do with T1D. I remember eating croissants every morning, seeing a total eclipse of the sun, enjoying great food, drinking wine, and living my life.

Life with diabetes hasn't always been easy for me, and like you, I've had my share of challenges.

I can remember many times when I wondered whether diabetes was going to hold me back. But I've always walked away from those challenging times with the confidence that I *can* handle it.

In the years following my diagnosis, I searched for information and tools to help me deal with the emotional roller coaster of life with T1D, and I always came up short. So, I decided to become a diabetes psychologist and create the resources and tools that would have been so helpful to me.

You Are Normal

If there is only one thing you take away from this book, I want you to know that you are normal.

No matter how T1D makes you feel, and no matter how much you are struggling right now, there is nothing wrong with you. Your experience is normal, even all of your uncomfortable thoughts and feelings about T1D.

Everyone with T1D has challenges. And if someone tells you they don't, they are either blissfully ignorant of the realities of life with diabetes or they're lying.

T1D is a sometimes-unpredictable medical condition that requires constant care and feeding. Trust me when I tell you uncomfortable thoughts and feelings are a normal reaction to the burden of diabetes.

I don't want anyone to have these types of feelings because of diabetes. But I also can't tell you with a straight face and a clear conscience that you'll never feel this way. If you do struggle with T1D, you are not doing anything wrong, and it is nothing to be ashamed of. Whatever you're feeling is simply a sign that you're human, and this is how humans respond to stressful situations.

Realizing that the emotional burden of T1D is normal was a big lesson for me. For many years after I was diagnosed with diabetes, I didn't know anyone else with it. And whenever I saw someone who had T1D, it was like spotting a rare, mystical creature in the wild.

DR. MARK'S T1D

As I was finishing grad school, I had a lot of challenges with diabetes. My blood sugars were nowhere near where I wanted them to be, and my frustration level was increasing every day. To make matters worse, I thought I should be able to cope with the rough parts of diabetes. I was studying to be a psychologist, after all. I remember feeling like I was the only person in the world with T1D who was struggling, and that was a lonely place to be.

One day, I had a severe low that really shook me up. When my blood sugar finally came up, I was confused, weak, and terrified. I was convinced that I was the only one this happened to, and I felt positive that nobody could ever understand what it felt like to have a blood sugar that low. I felt like the odd man out.

Not long afterward, something happened that changed my life. I was at the gym, and a woman about my age came up and said, "You have diabetes!" Caught off guard and wondering if I was talking to a psychic, I nodded yes. Then I saw her pointing at my pump site visible on my abdomen. During that brief interaction and our conversations at the gym in the weeks and months that followed, I realized that everything I was feeling and going through was normal. She told me about some of her experiences, and, for the first time, I found out I was not the only one who felt this way. I learned that even though my experience with T1D was not fun, it was normal.

And finding I was not alone in my struggles with T1D was a game-changer.

Quick note ───────────────────────

Just because your experiences and emotions are normal doesn't mean you don't want them to change. It doesn't mean you shouldn't work to make things easier for yourself. When I tell you that your experience with T1D is normal, all I'm saying is that anyone else in your situation would have a similar reaction. Your goal is to change your response to T1D. You might even say when T1D gets easier for you (and it will), your experiences and emotions will no longer be like everyone else's. They will be abnormal—and in this case, abnormal is good.

My Approach

As a diabetes psychologist, my approach to helping people navigate the emotional challenges of living with T1D is simple. It starts with being honest about how difficult life with T1D can sometimes be. I have found it does nobody any good to sugarcoat these facts.

I think it is helpful to be honest, even blunt, about the challenges of T1D for one simple reason: If you are not truthful about the impact T1D has on your life, you cannot take steps to change it.

There is no easy fix for the emotional challenges of T1D. Sometimes, people want to find that one thing they can do differently that will simplify T1D and make them feel better. You may be looking for that thing in this book.

Spoiler alert! It doesn't exist. And the more time spent looking for a magical solution, the more stressful life with T1D becomes. This approach makes sense on paper. However, it just doesn't work.

I don't think it's possible to eliminate the burden of T1D in your life completely. But I also don't think this means all hope is lost—quite the opposite. My approach is to help you learn how to navigate around the stress of T1D, so it doesn't hold you back. When you can do this, the emotional burden of T1D may be annoying, but it is no longer devastating.

What This Book Is About

In this book, I'm going to show you how to navigate the emotional challenges of T1D, walking you through the process step by step. But first, you have to acknowledge that diabetes sucks. Only then can you take the steps to deal with it.

This book is not a magic bullet. You will not be able to read it and expect all the stress of T1D to disappear without any work on your part. The strategies you'll learn are effective, but you have to put in the effort if you want to see results. You have to work to become the person who can handle whatever T1D throws your way.

This book is about taking action to deal with the cards you have been dealt. You won't find a pity party here. You will find an acknowledgment of the reality of life with T1D and the encouragement, support, and tools you need to live the best life possible in the context of this reality.

Here is a preview of what you'll find in this book:

Chapter 1 talks about what it means to handle T1D.

Chapters 2, 3, and 4 are about why you have to be honest with yourself about the challenges of T1D and what they look like (and don't look like) in your life.

Chapter 5 talks about why trying to control your emotional experience with T1D almost always backfires.

Chapter 6 discusses why putting in the work to manage T1D is critical to handling it even when you don't want to.

Chapter 7 is about how to deal with the uncomfortable emotions that come with T1D.

Chapter 8 shows how taking action, even when you're scared, helps you handle T1D.

Chapter 9 talks about why getting support from other people is vital.

Chapter 10 prepares you to handle some of the significant curveballs T1D throws your way.

Chapter 11 helps you decide when you need professional help.

Chapter 12 shows you how to go beyond handling T1D and thrive.

How To Use This Book

This book is meant to be a resource you can come back to over and over. I recommend reading it all the way through the first time, and then referring to specific sections when you need them. Reading it in its entirety once will give you the context you need to get the most out of it as a resource.

If you feel overwhelmed and are looking for skills you can use today, skip ahead to Chapter 7. But be sure to flip back and read the beginning of the book once you are feeling steadier on your feet.

Throughout the book, there are exercises to help put the concepts into action. If you find them helpful, do them. If not, skip them!

You'll also find stories to illustrate the challenges people with T1D face on a daily basis. All the stories are based on real people who live with T1D. However, their names and some identifying details have been changed. I also included stories about my life with T1D to show that even though

I do this for a living, I still experience many of the same challenges as you.

Who Is This Book For? (And who isn't it for?)

You may wonder if this book is right for you and if you will get any value from reading it. Here is the answer:

- *If T1D has left you overwhelmed, burned out, and at your wit's end, then this book is for you.*

- *If you find diabetes tolerable but irritating and are looking for better ways to deal with it, then this book is for you.*

- *If you're doing okay right now, but have had trouble dealing with T1D in the past, then this book is for you.*

- *If you are newly diagnosed and want to make sure you have all the tools necessary to handle the stress T1D will bring in the future, this book is for you.*

- *If you love someone who lives with T1D and want to understand what they are dealing with and how you can support them, then this book is for you.*

- *If you're a diabetes rock star who has never experienced any emotional challenges with T1D and you are confident T1D will never be stressful for you, this book is **NOT** for you.*

Handling T1D starts right here, right now. Let's get to it!

Chapter 1

YOU CAN HANDLE THE STRESS OF T1D

IT ALWAYS SEEMS
IMPOSSIBLE UNTIL IT'S DONE.

—NELSON MANDELA

CLOSE YOUR EYES. Picture yourself three months from now.

Nothing about T1D has changed for you. Your blood sugars are still wacky. The mental gymnastics are still stressful. A cloud of burnout still casts a shadow over your life.

T1D still sucks.

But one thing has changed—your ability to handle it.

You are moving through your life with new confidence. The emotional burden of T1D doesn't faze you because you know what to expect and how to get through it. When the stress of diabetes burnout starts to creep in, you take note of it, but don't let it stop you from living life.

When you know you can handle T1D, guess what happens?

T1D becomes so much less of a big deal.

I know you are not there yet.

I know you may not think this type of freedom is possible with T1D. Right now, you're still having a hard time dealing with the everyday pressure of T1D. Minor annoyances become a big deal. You probably have a hard time believing it will ever be possible to handle everything diabetes throws your way. And you certainly cannot imagine being able to manage T1D with confidence, handling the bumps in the road, no matter how big.

I know how impossible this can seem.

Almost everyone I have worked with over the past ten years has had the same challenges. On the surface, each person's struggles with T1D look a little different, but they all fall into the same general category. Almost all are having a hard time handling the stressful parts of T1D.

Diabetes makes them feel overwhelmed, burned out, anxious, or some other combination of uncomfortable emotions.

Everyone wants to find a better way to deal with their diabetes-related emotions so that they stop getting in their way.

I have some good news.

Over the past ten years, I haven't met one person who hasn't been able to handle the emotional burden of T1D.

Right now, you may be thinking you're going to be the exception. You will be that one person who won't be able to deal with the stress of T1D. But don't worry! You are not alone. Most people struggling with T1D come to a point where they start to doubt that they'll be able to handle it. They beat themselves up because they think they should be having an easier time with diabetes.

Then other thoughts start creeping in. Thoughts such as…

- *If I'm having a hard time dealing with the minor inconveniences of diabetes, how on earth will I be able to deal with the big stuff?*

- *Diabetes has worn me down and has taken away my ability to handle stress.*

- *I'm just not cut out for all the pressure of T1D.*

- *T1D sucks, and I can't handle it.*

As you read this book, let me ask that you do one thing.

It is the same thing I've asked every patient over the years. If you are willing to humor this request, I'm confident you're more than halfway to being able to handle T1D. Ready?

Here it is…

Be open to the possibility that you'll be able to handle T1D.

I have met so many people—including maybe you—who believe they cannot handle the emotional burden of T1D.

You have tried so many times and have failed just as many. Every time you think your feet are firmly planted on the ground, T1D rattles you, and you lose your proverbial balance and fall.

Pretty soon, you start to think you'll never be able to get on solid ground with your diabetes. The emotional burden will always be too much to handle, and there's no chance it can ever be different.

If you're having a hard time coping with T1D, there is probably a part of you that wonders whether you'll ever be able to handle the pressure. Through my work, I have met many folks in your shoes, and they have taught me something simple yet profound.

The minute you doubt that you can handle T1D, you will have a hard time dealing with it. Once you start believing you can't cope, you trap yourself and seal your fate. You won't be able to handle it.

You must be open to the possibility that dealing with the stress of T1D is possible.

What Handling T1D Looks Like

You may be wondering what it means to handle T1D, and more importantly, how you will know when you are doing so?

I want to set you up for success and describe what it means to handle T1D. Once you see what "handling it" looks like in real life (and what it doesn't look like), you will start to see how it might be possible to get there.

Handling T1D is not some magical place you arrive at where life with diabetes is easy and you never have negative feelings. It's the opposite. To handle T1D means recognizing that it sucks—that it is emotionally taxing and physically exhausting—and knowing you have what it takes to carry it with you and not let it get in your way.

WHEN YOU CAN HANDLE T1D...
You are willing to be uncomfortable and take action anyway.

This is a tough one. Being able to handle stress does not mean that the emotional burden of T1D will go away. It is not some peaceful place where life with T1D is easy. It may be the opposite. It is possible that when you get to a place where you feel like you can deal with it, nothing about life with T1D will have changed for you on the outside. Your blood sugar roller coasters may still be there. You may still feel overwhelmed and burned out. Your devices may still embarrass you. Handling T1D has nothing to do with how you feel and everything to do with how you behave.

Handling T1D means acknowledging that diabetes sucks, that it is uncomfortable, and choosing not to let it get in your way. It means being willing to tolerate the parts of diabetes that aren't very much fun so you can do what you want to do.

REAL-LIFE T1D: BRINTON
Brinton was terrified to take more than three units of insulin at a time. Anytime she entered carbs into her pump, and it suggested she bolus more than three

units, her anxiety took off. Her heart started beating quickly, her mind raced, and she had to sit down. Brinton loved cooking and baking, and she loved to eat. But with her fear of taking what most people would consider an average-size bolus, her blood sugar was high most of the time—her last A1c was over 9%.

I saw Brinton for several sessions, and we worked to help her see that she would continue with this same behavior until she was able to trust her judgment, body, basal rates, and insulin-to-carb ratios. She told me she understood but continued to hesitate to make changes.

One week, Brinton showed up at my office with a big smile on her face. The night before, she had gone out to dinner with her boyfriend, and when the server put the pasta in front of her, she pulled out her pump and bolused almost eight units. As she went on to tell me all about her dinner, I stopped her and asked what happened to her anxiety.

She told me she felt extremely anxious giving herself that big (for her) bolus. But she decided she could be anxious and still trust herself. I asked her what happened after she gave herself the insulin.

She smiled and said, "I had a lovely dinner with my boyfriend. I'll admit I was a little nervous, but I can feel anxious and not let those feelings get to me."

WHEN YOU CAN HANDLE T1D...
You respond with grace to the curveballs T1D throws you.

One thing I know for sure about T1D is that it can be unpredictable. You can do the same thing every day and get different results each time. Diabetes is not always going to make sense. That's just the way it is, and that is a big part of what makes diabetes so stressful.

When you're able to handle T1D, you respond to these challenges with grace. You notice them, and you do everything in your power to deal with them. But you don't let these situations get to you, even when you swing at them and miss.

Responding to the challenges of T1D with grace means coming to a place where you can accept that there may not be much you can do to control them or prevent them from happening. It also means being aware of what you do have control over and taking intentional steps to influence the outcome. You can acknowledge that these unexpected situations aren't fun to deal with while remembering you get to choose how to respond to them.

When you respond to the T1D curveballs with grace, the stress of T1D becomes easier to handle.

WHEN YOU CAN HANDLE T1D...
You don't let the challenging parts of T1D get in your way.

Handling T1D means being able to separate what you feel from how you behave. Diabetes can bring on some uncomfortable emotions, but you know your discomfort doesn't have to control your behavior. You can do what you want to do, even when it's stressful. You can accept that T1D is challenging, but these challenges don't have to prevent you from doing what you want to do. Navigating the challenging emotions that come with T1D may take some effort, but these emotions are no longer a barrier that prevent you from taking action.

How many times have you told yourself that you can't do something because of how T1D makes you feel?

For example...

- *I can't take the full bolus for my food because I'm scared of going low.*

- *I can't go to the zoo with my kids because I'm over-whelmed with diabetes.*

- *I can't wear my continuous glucose monitor (CGM) out to the bar because people will ask me what it is, and I'll be embarrassed.*

This way of thinking makes you believe you have to choose between taking action in your life and dealing with diabetes.

You tell yourself that you can't handle the challenges of diabetes. And because you think you can't handle it, you take steps to avoid the stress instead of dealing with it.

Handling diabetes doesn't mean you avoid it—quite the opposite. It means allowing the uncomfortable feelings to be there and not letting them stop you from living your life.

Handling T1D means living your life, even though the stress is along for the ride.

WHEN YOU CAN HANDLE T1D...
You stay present.

You can only deal with the stress of T1D in the present moment. Handling T1D means dealing with it as it comes instead of letting your mind wander to the past or jump to the future. Guilt about the past and worry about the future make diabetes even more difficult to handle than it already is. Staying present helps you handle whatever emotions you are experiencing.

REAL-LIFE T1D: LUCY

"Diabetes sucks. But that's okay. I got it."

Ever since her diagnosis three years ago, this has been Lucy's mantra. She doesn't try to make diabetes anything more or anything less than what it is. And a lot of the time, T1D is a pain in Lucy's behind. As a nurse, she worries about her blood sugar during her twelve-hour shifts. As a twenty-eight-year-old woman who dreams of getting married, Lucy worries her CGM will make her less attractive to the men she dates. Sometimes, late at night, she finds herself awake in bed, asking what she did to deserve the emotional burden of T1D. But no matter what, Lucy always comes back to her mantra.

Lucy knows she can handle T1D by acknowledging it and moving forward.

REAL-LIFE T1D: DAVID

For a long time, David did everything he could think

of to control the stress of diabetes. Nothing worked.

He tried ignoring diabetes. He tried planning every detail of his day. He tried keeping a rigid routine that he never deviated from. None of these strategies helped, at least in the long run.

One day, something clicked for David. He was playing golf, and his blood sugar dropped suddenly, something he always worked hard to avoid. To his surprise, he treated his low and was able to continue his round.

He discovered he could handle the emotional burden of diabetes by letting his guard down because he wasn't always waiting for T1D to come and get him. David accepted what he could not control with T1D and found that was the key to his success.

What Handling T1D Doesn't Mean

When I suggest that people can handle the emotional burden of type 1 diabetes, the most common response is confusion and pushback.

Handing the stress of T1D is not the solution they are looking for. They want to get rid of it.

There is a lot of confusion about what it means to handle T1D, and I want to clear up some of that confusion.

HANDLING T1D DOESN'T MEAN...
You love T1D or that you want it in your life.

I have never met anyone who wants to have T1D or who wouldn't give it away in a heartbeat if that were possible.

Handling T1D means coming to a place of acceptance, not attraction. It means being okay with having T1D around, not running toward it with open arms.

REAL-LIFE T1D: JENNY

Jenny couldn't fathom being in a place where she wanted to have T1D. Since her diagnosis four years ago, diabetes has done nothing but get in her way. In her mind, T1D has taken away her spontaneity, self-confidence, and dreams for the future. She thought being willing to handle the stress of T1D would make all the downsides of living with T1D even worse. Once she reframed how she thought about T1D and saw that being willing to handle diabetes and loving it are not the same thing, her mind opened to the possibility that she could handle it.

HANDLING T1D DOESN'T MEAN...
You have to enjoy anything about type 1 diabetes.

Some people worry that if they can handle T1D, this will mean that T1D will become enjoyable. They see this as an impossible task (and to be honest, it probably is), so they don't even consider the possibility of trying to deal with it. Handling T1D doesn't mean working toward enjoying it. It means being aware that you will not enjoy it most of the time and working to be okay with this reality. Things you enjoy are easy to handle. But you also can handle things you don't like, including T1D. It just takes some work.

HANDLING T1D DOESN'T MEAN...
You are perfect at managing T1D.

Handling T1D does not mean living in a utopian fantasy world where your blood sugars are perfect all the time. Instead, it means knowing your management is never going to be perfect and being okay with that. You are going to have challenges, and your goal is to develop skills to navigate these challenges. You can deal with whatever T1D throws at you and come out the other side no worse for the wear.

DR. MARK'S T1D

After lots of work, I think I handle T1D pretty well. But I'll be honest with you. My diabetes management is far from perfect. Just like you, I have blood sugar swings. I go low at the worst times. I don't always make the best food choices, and I don't always count my carbs correctly (or sometimes at all). I forget to bolus more often than I want to admit. I have to tell you, though, I can handle the stress of diabetes because I am not perfect. I am okay with the imperfections in my diabetes management, and I know that's a big reason why I'm able to handle it.

Why Bother?
You may be thinking to yourself, *this all sounds great, but it also sounds like a lot of hard work.*

I get it! You're used to running away from T1D, and handling diabetes means leaning into the challenges. In theory, you understand why trying to handle T1D is a good idea, but you wonder if doing the hard work will be worth it.

I know the answer is yes.

I know the work is worth it because I have seen so many people thrive with T1D once they see they can handle it. It is undoubtedly worth it, and I know you will agree when you give it a try.

You get to choose whether you are willing to put in the work. I'm here to guide you, but I can't force you to do it. What I can do is tell you about what life can be like for you when you can handle T1D.

WHEN YOU CAN HANDLE T1D...
You'll have more freedom and flexibility in your life.

Close your eyes and imagine what life would be like if T1D didn't hold you back. You have the freedom to do whatever you want, and diabetes is just there in the background.

Do you want to go on a spontaneous road trip? *Then go!*

Do you want to have that extra piece of pizza and an ice cream sundae? *Then eat both!*

Do you want to wear that tank top and let the world see your CGM? *Diabetes doesn't even come into the equation when you decide what to wear.*

When you can handle T1D, freedom and flexibility follow close behind. Diabetes is still with you, but it doesn't keep you trapped. You can do whatever you want with confidence and can handle the annoyances and inconveniences of diabetes along the way.

WHEN YOU CAN HANDLE T1D...

T1D stops getting in the way of your life.

The emotional burden of diabetes can be a barrier to doing the things you want to do in your life. It can feel like a weight on your shoulders that holds you back. Handling T1D means not letting the stress of T1D stand in your way.

REAL-LIFE T1D: WINONA

Winona's biggest complaint about diabetes is she feels like it always stands between her and her dreams, both big and small. She wants to date, but she is worried nobody will want to be with her when they see the diabetes devices she wears on her body. Winona wants to take up surfing, but thinking about managing her blood sugar in the water is overwhelming and stops her before she even gets started. And her biggest dream is to be a mother, but the thought of being pregnant with T1D stops her in her tracks.

The emotional burden of T1D is getting in Winona's way. Then she worries that she won't be able to handle this pressure, which makes T1D even more stressful.

If she can roll with the stress and handle it, Winona would be in a much better place. Diabetes will no longer get in her way because she will be confident she can handle it. Her thoughts and fears will still be there, but they won't stop her from doing anything. They will simply be bumps in the road and not the massive roadblocks that have been there in the past.

WHEN YOU CAN HANDLE T1D...
The challenges become less of a big deal.

When you are confident you can handle the challenging parts of diabetes, they become easier to navigate. No, it doesn't make them go away, but they become easier to face. There is freedom and flexibility in handling the stress because you are willing to lean into it.

REAL-LIFE T1D: JOHN

If John could spend every day doing just one thing, he would break dance. It is truly his passion. He has been dancing since he was a young teen, and his T1D diagnosis at age seventeen didn't stop him.

In his mid-twenties, things changed for John. He felt like he had to choose between diabetes and break dancing. John's doctor was pushing him toward using an insulin pump and CGM, and he could not imagine how he could wear these devices while dancing. He started to see break dancing and managing T1D as incompatible, and so John chose break dancing.

Once he made the choice, he started feeling much more anxious about his diabetes and his health in general. Every time John's blood sugar rose, he was overwhelmed with thoughts about the damage he was doing to his body. But instead of trying to figure out how to manage his blood sugar while break dancing, John pushed on, stuck in his belief that he had to sacrifice his future health to keep doing what brought him joy.

After we started working together, John told me he was willing to push himself and see if he could manage his diabetes while break dancing—and he surprised himself. He pushed himself to see what break dancing with a CGM was like. John discovered the CGM didn't get in his way, and he could dance even better because his blood sugars were in range. He tried something new, which allowed him to get unstuck from his either-or way of thinking. John had the evidence he needed that he could handle break dancing and T1D at the same time.

WHEN YOU CAN HANDLE T1D...
You'll be able to start seeing the positives.

Knowing you can handle T1D allows you to see the silver linings. When diabetes is a struggle you feel you can't handle, all you see are the challenges because they are always in your face. Confidence you can handle something also brings perspective. You can see the challenges but are also more open to seeing the positives diabetes brings to your life (and yes, there are some). But you have to be willing to experience the hard stuff to open your eyes to the positives, and leaning into T1D can open up a whole new world.

How I Know You Can Handle T1D
I know you may not believe me right now, but I am confident you can handle anything T1D throws your way. You have already been handling diabetes, even if you are unaware of it. Maybe you haven't dealt with it in the best way possible, and that's okay. There is always room for

improvement, and this book will show how you can handle the stress of T1D more effectively. But know that you have it in you to handle and thrive with T1D. All you have to do is to build on what you've already done.

Right now, you may not feel confident you can handle everything about T1D. However, I am sure you can do it. Here's why.

YOU CAN HANDLE T1D BECAUSE...
You have T1D.

You can handle T1D because you have T1D. I know this sounds like circular logic, but it isn't. Diabetes is demanding. It requires a lot from you. And you are doing it. You may not be perfect (spoiler alert—none of us are!), and it may not feel like you're doing a great job at handling it, but you're reading this book right now and looking for ways to improve yourself. That is a sign that you can handle T1D.

Feeling overwhelmed, and burned out are not signs that you can't handle T1D. The fact that you're still living your life and want to keep improving is strong evidence that you can handle the challenging parts of diabetes because that is exactly what you've been doing since being diagnosed.

YOU CAN HANDLE T1D BECAUSE...
You are strong.

I have never met anyone with T1D who isn't stronger in some way because of diabetes. You know that managing this condition day in and day out means always being on your toes. You have to make important decisions about your health, pivot your strategy regularly, and keep going, no matter what. You are already doing this.

Sometimes it may feel like you're not doing a perfect job, and, of course, there is always room for improvement. But the reality is T1D has made you stronger. You have to be resilient to survive with diabetes. The fact that you live with T1D proves you are strong. I hope you see it too.

Exercise

Take a minute and make a list of all the ways T1D has made you stronger and more resilient. Write down whatever comes to mind. Don't second-guess yourself or overthink it. Just write. You might be surprised at what you come up with.

YOU CAN HANDLE T1D BECAUSE...
You can do hard things.

I know you can handle the tricky parts of living with T1D because you can do difficult things. You live with diabetes, and that's challenging. That means you're already doing something really tough.

Let that sink in for a minute.

One of the biggest barriers to believing you can handle T1D is the belief that working to deal with it will be too difficult. You think somehow diabetes is more complicated than everything else in your life. Maybe for you, some parts of diabetes are more difficult than the other challenges you have in your life.

The best way to see you can handle diabetes is to remember you've been able to cope with difficult things in the past. Once you realize that you've been able to overcome similar challenges and emerge relatively unscathed on the other side, you'll know you can handle T1D, even though it's hard.

Exercise

Think beyond T1D for a minute. Write down some things you've done in your life that have been hard. These things can be big or small, recent or in the distant past. Think about what you have done at school or work, in your relationships, athletics, as a parent. You do hard things all the time—we all do.

When you finish writing this list, look it over, and pat yourself on the back. You can do difficult things because you've already done them. And since you can do hard things, I am positive you can lean in and handle the stress of T1D.

You'll Only Know if You Try

I know you can handle the tough stuff with T1D, but you still may be skeptical. You may not even believe me, and that's okay. I don't expect you to believe me without doing your own research and coming to your own conclusions.

So how do you gather the evidence you need so you can see for yourself whether you can handle diabetes, even though it sucks? The short answer is, you will never know unless you try.

Allow Yourself the Opportunity to Find Out

You will never know whether you can handle the stress of T1D unless you try. I want to challenge you to trust yourself and trust the process that I am going to lay out so you can see what is possible. Think about what will happen if you never allow yourself the opportunity to handle it. You will have failed before you even started, and you'll stay stuck right where you are. And my guess is, that's not where you want to stay.

Try to Trust Me and My Experience

I know this may be hard, but try to trust that I know what I'm talking about. I've worked with hundreds of people with T1D who have been exactly where you are right now. They felt stuck, like T1D was holding them back. They were having trouble coming to terms with the fact that T1D sucks. Like you, they had convinced themselves that things could never get better because they thought they couldn't handle diabetes.

Right now, most of these folks are in a much better place with T1D. By following the process, there is no reason you will not be in this better place soon too.

Handling Diabetes Is a Skill

You may be thinking to yourself that if you could handle diabetes, you would already be doing it. You may be worried that because you haven't figured it out yet, you're not capable of handling the pressure, and even trying is a lost cause. Nothing could be further from the truth.

Handling the emotional burden of T1D requires learning a set of skills. These skills require practice and don't always come naturally. If you're having trouble handling T1D now, all it means is you just haven't learned the right set of skills yet.

Identify the Person You Need to Become

As you read on, keep the following question in mind.

Who is the person you need to become to handle the stress of living with T1D?

Handling T1D may mean pushing yourself into unfamiliar places. Growing in this way involves more than just checking a box and doing new things. It means growing into a new person—one who can deal with the reality that T1D sucks but doesn't let this hard truth get in their way.

Do you need to become more patient? More flexible? Do you need to become more focused on the details or more mindful?

The possibilities are endless, and only you can identify the person you need to become to be able to handle, and maybe even thrive, with and despite the stress of T1D.

Think about What Happens if You Don't Try

I know this process feels scary. I also know that you are struggling right now, and you want something to change. The only way to change is to take action. I know you can do difficult things for sure because you do hard things every day. All I am asking you to do is commit to trying. I think you may be surprised at what you're capable of.

The process of learning how to handle T1D begins in an unlikely place.

It starts by being honest with yourself about how much T1D sucks.

—————— **CHAPTER 1 KEY TAKEAWAYS** ——————

- *Get out of your own way. The first step to handling T1D is being open to the possibility you might be able to handle it.*

- *Handling T1D does not mean life is going to be easy. It means you can deal with the challenges when they come—and they will.*

- *Handling T1D means living your life, even though stress is along for the ride.*

- *When you can handle T1D, your life gets better, even though you still have diabetes and it is still hard.*

- *You have already proven to yourself you can do difficult things (after all, you live with T1D), so you can handle whatever T1D throws your way. You may not believe that right now, but stay open to the possibility.*

Chapter 2

HONESTY IS THE BEST POLICY

HONESTY IS THE FIRST CHAPTER
IN THE BOOK OF WISDOM.

—THOMAS JEFFERSON

I WOULD BE willing to bet that you are not completely honest with yourself about your experience with type 1 diabetes.

You are not lying to yourself on purpose. If you're like most people with T1D (including me), you've probably just slipped into some patterns of thinking that are not entirely accurate. But just because this happens to most people doesn't mean it's helpful.

The first and most important step to handling the stress of T1D is being brutally honest with yourself about what it's like to live with diabetes. You're not doing yourself any favors by not being truthful about life with T1D, including the struggles.

Let's start with a couple of simple facts.

If you're not honest with yourself about the challenges you're having with T1D, there's no way you'll be able to handle them. The first step to dealing with something is admitting that it's there.

- *You have to give the challenge a name.*

- *You have to feel the discomfort that it brings about.*

- *You have to be willing to sit with that discomfort to understand how it is affecting you.*

To start, you have to identify the things about T1D that are hard for you. Name them. Look at the challenging aspects of T1D in the face and describe them. The more specific you can be, the better.

When you name your challenges, you make them real so you can confront them. I know this sounds scary, but being honest about your challenges and facing them head-on is the only way to start handling them. If you're not willing to admit they are causing problems in your life, you're going to stay stuck feeling overwhelmed with nothing to grab onto and nothing specific to work toward.

Even worse, when you minimize the challenges you're having, you ignore the reality of your experience—and sometimes the reality is that T1D sucks.

REAL-LIFE T1D: EMILY

As Emily put the key in her office door, she plastered a smile on her face and repeated her usual mantra.

The words, "I'm doing just great, and it's going to be a great day," played on repeat in her mind, trying to drown out the noise of her CGM alarm going off every five minutes. The truth is, Emily wasn't anywhere close to doing great. A blood sugar roller coaster had kept her awake all night. Exhausted and angry, she saw her calendar full of meetings that day. She had to get through it. Reality be damned, she thought. "Diabetes just isn't that hard, and it certainly is not going to ruin my day," she whispered under her breath.

Emily dismisses the challenges of T1D to herself and other people every day. She doesn't see any other option to get diabetes out of her way. Emily figures if she just tells herself and everybody else that it's not that big of a deal, then maybe eventually it won't be. Then, when diabetes gets challenging, her guilt piles on because she thinks she shouldn't be feeling this way.

Emily feels like she's living a double life. There's the life she tells herself she has with T1D and the one she is experiencing while pretending it's not there.

But honesty works both ways. You may minimize how hard T1D is, but you also can exaggerate it at times.

When you exaggerate the challenges of living with T1D, you are not being honest with yourself. You let the real challenges you're experiencing snowball. Your mind takes an objectively stressful situation—but one you can handle—and twists it into something that anybody would have a hard time dealing with. When you do this (and we all do it sometimes), you're not being fair to yourself.

We exaggerate our experiences with T1D in big and small ways all the time. I know I do.

DR. MARK'S T1D

I always have my insulin pump in my pocket, and the tubing is often peeking out the top. When I'm running around the kitchen cooking dinner, it's not uncommon for the tubing to get caught on a cabinet or drawer and pull me back, like I'm on a leash. It happens; it's annoying. But objectively, it's just not that big of a deal. The best-case scenario is I get a little pull at my infusion site. The worst-case scenario is the entire site gets pulled out, and I have to take a break from cooking and spend a couple of minutes changing it.

Irritating? Yes!

Catastrophic? Not in the slightest.

But when I feel that tug in the moment, especially when it happens more than once in a short period, I get so angry. I get mad at myself, at my pump, and at diabetes. The situation usually snowballs, and I go down a rabbit hole thinking about all the extra challenges I have because of T1D. And it doesn't help when my wife sees the tubing get caught and gasps, making anyone around us think the kitchen is on fire.

I'll be the first to admit that I am not being completely honest with myself about diabetes in those moments. Instead, I take a legitimate challenge, and my mind makes it much more dramatic than it needs to be—all for no good reason.

Reasons You Aren't Honest with Yourself

Hopefully, you are starting to see why being honest with yourself is such an essential part of seeing you can handle T1D.

You may have even thought of some areas in your life with diabetes where you have not been completely honest with yourself. That's great! As we'll talk about later in this chapter, pinpointing where you are not truthful with yourself is the first step to becoming more honest.

Before we get there, let's take a closer look at some of the reasons you may be having a hard time being honest with yourself about how the stress of T1D impacts or doesn't impact your life. After all, if honesty were easy, you probably would be doing it more already.

How would things change if you were completely honest with yourself about how much T1D sucks?

This is a blunt and hard-hitting, but necessary, question to ask yourself.

If you are completely honest with yourself about how the emotional burden of T1D affects you, you may not like what you see. Honesty means accepting that you have a chronic condition. It also means acknowledging that you have an extra burden in your day-to-day life that most others don't have to deal with. It means admitting that T1D can make you feel frustrated, anxious, burned out, and even hopeless sometimes.

Let's be honest. That is what T1D can feel like. It's not fun. Opening that door and letting those feelings in is not pleasant.

Sometimes it's easier to just brush over these experiences. But ignoring the stress does nothing to change the reality of what you're feeling. Pretending like you aren't having a hard time is not exactly honest.

When I suggest that people sometimes exaggerate the difficulties of T1D, a lot of people get defensive. They respond with...

"How dare you suggest that diabetes is not as challenging as I say it is!"

I gently remind them I'm not trying to minimize how much T1D sucks. But I do want them to be honest with themselves about their challenges so they can lean into the real ones and let go of the others.

When you feel overwhelmed with T1D—and most of us do at times—your brain tries to make sense of these feelings. Your emotions give you a signal that something is not right. You may be in danger, and you may have to react. You tend to jump to the most extreme end first, so you are prepared for the worst, and then you can pull back and see things more realistically once you get your bearings. The challenge is, it's easy to get stuck at the extreme end, especially when you can't make sense of what you are feeling and why.

Then the next time something stressful with T1D comes along—a low blood sugar, an occlusion, your CGM screaming at you, an ignorant comment—you go back to that same place, a place that doesn't reflect the reality of the situation. When you make those minor stresses a big deal, you start having difficulty believing you can handle them.

REAL-LIFE T1D: LEE

From the minute Lee's boyfriend invited her to go with his family to their lake house, her mind jumped to how she could hide her diabetes. They would be spending most days at the lake on their boat, which means Lee would have to manage T1D out in the open.

Lee has always been self-conscious about her diabetes, but this was different. This new relationship was off to a good start. Her boyfriend was supportive, caring, and they had so much fun together. On their second date, she built up the courage to tell him about T1D, and he didn't even blink an eye. She so badly wanted to make a good impression on his parents, and she was worried about how they would react when they found out she has T1D. Lee's mind was consumed with how she would play it cool if they saw her check her blood sugar on the boat. She even considered taking a break from checking her blood sugar and taking insulin when she was on the boat so she wouldn't have to bring it up.

Lee was terrified her boyfriend's parents would see her as broken and not good enough to date her son. Then Lee worried their opinion might rub off on her

*boyfriend, and he would go along with whatever his
parents thought about her. She got herself so worked
up she seriously considered telling her boyfriend she
had a deadline at work and that her boss told her she
couldn't take that week off.*

Notice how Lee took a situation that anyone would consider stressful, and made it into a much bigger deal. She let her mind snowball to the worst possible outcome and then spent excessive energy trying to figure out how she could avoid this unlikely situation.

I have to wonder how much easier it would have been if Lee had taken a step back and was honest with herself about the real challenges she was facing and what the likely outcome would be. My guess is this injection of honesty would have been refreshing and opened her eyes to the fact that she could handle her boyfriend's parents, no matter how they reacted to her diabetes.

Honesty Sets You Up for Success

When you are honest with yourself about the challenges of T1D, you set yourself up for success. I know it's not easy to admit that you are struggling with diabetes. Or maybe you have told yourself you're having a hard time, but you have avoided identifying the real reasons diabetes is so challenging for you.

When you're honest about why you're having a rough time with diabetes, you open yourself up to vulnerability. But you also empower yourself to take charge of the situation.

Honesty means looking in the mirror and facing the struggles you're having with T1D. It means giving them a name. It also means looking closely at how these struggles are impacting your life.

Examining your experience in this way can be scary, but when you have a clear view of what is going on, you can take steps to make changes. Being honest with yourself about how hard T1D is helps set you up for success.

On the flip side, being honest and calling yourself out when you're making the challenges of T1D bigger than they actually are also sets you up for success. There's absolutely no reason to make life with diabetes any harder than it has to be. When you can see the emotional burden of diabetes for what it is, you make it easier to handle, which exponentially increases the chance you will be successful. Without being honest and reining in your thoughts, handling the stress probably feels more like a fleeting wish than something you can achieve.

REAL-LIFE T1D: JOEL

After Joel was diagnosed with T1D, he thought his life was over. Leaving his doctor's office with a list of things he had to do to manage diabetes, he felt confused and overwhelmed. Joel had no idea how he was going to get through the next week of this new normal, let alone the rest of his life. He was 44 years old, and he thought the diagnosis meant he would be stuck at home for the rest of his life.

Before his diagnosis, Joel lived an active life. He went on weekend fishing trips, rode his motorcycle, and loved camping with his wife and their dogs. Now seven years later, he hasn't done any of those things. Diabetes is overwhelming for Joel, and he doesn't want to even think about rocking the boat.

The first time I talked to Joel, he told me how much he missed his old life. I asked him why he hadn't been out on his motorcycle or camping since his diagnosis, and he looked at me like I was crazy. He told me that doing these things would just make T1D even worse for him. I challenged Joel to be honest with himself about the emotional strain of T1D.

With some work, Joel was able to see that even though diabetes made him feel overwhelmed at times, he was not being honest with himself about his ability to handle this stress. Yes, it was there, but it was not as overwhelming as he was making it out to be. Camping, fishing, and riding his motorcycle with T1D will take a bit of planning, but it's nothing he can't deal with. Once he was honest with himself about how stressful these things would be (or, in this case, not be), Joel's world opened up. Looking inward and being honest with himself set Joel up for success.

Not Being Honest Sets You Up for Failure

When you are not honest with yourself about T1D, dealing effectively with the challenges diabetes brings with it becomes nearly impossible. Without honesty, you do not even allow yourself the opportunity to handle it.

One story I hear repeatedly is how people try to pretend they don't have diabetes. They figure if they ignore diabetes long enough, it will just disappear. So they don't check their blood sugar, take insulin, or even think about diabetes. This strategy usually makes them feel better for a very short time. But you can guess how the story ends. Instead of making T1D easier, ignoring it always comes back to bite them in the rear, making their life more about diabetes, not less.

Sugarcoating life with T1D and not acknowledging the challenges it brings means ignoring and avoiding your true feelings and experiences. You may be able to sidestep feeling burned out or overwhelmed by diabetes momentarily, but in the end, you make T1D even more stressful. Your dishonesty backfires.

Ignoring the fact you have T1D simply doesn't work, and neither does glossing over the fact that you are struggling with diabetes. Pretending like you're not having a hard time doesn't mean you're not having a hard time. When you don't acknowledge that you're struggling, you don't allow yourself the opportunity to deal with the challenges. They fester under the surface, and they get more ingrained. Over time, the skills you use to deal with them get rusty.

On the other end of the spectrum, when you take the stress of T1D and make it worse than it actually is, you also set yourself up for failure. The human mind can quickly spiral to a worst-case scenario with T1D. The further your mind spirals, the more difficult diabetes gets, and the harder it is to bring your experience back to reality. Your patterns of thinking get ingrained and make you believe that diabetes really is that difficult. The further you let your thoughts spiral without checking them, the more you set yourself up for failure.

Honesty Is the Best Policy

The best way to handle the stress of T1D is to be honest with yourself about it.

What is your first thought when reading the following statements?

- *Living with T1D is not that hard. It's really not that big of a deal. Diabetes never gets in my way and has absolutely no impact on my life. T1D is easy.*

- *Living with T1D is impossible. It is so overwhelming that I cannot live a normal life. I am constantly stressed out, and I have to pay attention to my blood sugars or disaster will strike. I hate T1D.*

It's unlikely that either of these statements is entirely accurate. There may be kernels of truth in each, but the reality is probably somewhere in the middle. No, T1D is not easy, but it's nowhere near impossible.

When you uncover the reality of your experience with T1D, and you're honest with yourself about what this experience looks like for you, you'll be in a much better place to successfully deal with whatever challenges T1D puts in your path.

Honesty Is Hard

If being honest with yourself about the reality of living with T1D were easy, you probably would have done it by now.

But there are several reasons why being honest about T1D is not easy.

First, honesty means acknowledging how you are doing right now. It means accepting you have T1D, that managing it takes work, and that diabetes may be wearing you down, both mentally and physically. These truths can be a hard pill to swallow.

Taking an honest look at T1D also may mean you have to admit you've been wrong and that T1D is a lot more doable than you've made it out to be. It may mean admitting that you've been making things harder on yourself than they needed to be. Admitting you're wrong is never easy, especially when it means your experience with T1D did not need to be so difficult.

Exercise

Here are some steps you can take to make sure you are as honest with yourself as possible about your life with T1D.

1. Commit to being honest. Honestly, it is never easy, especially when it means admitting you are not doing great or accepting that your way of thinking was inaccurate. Taking steps to be honest with yourself means being willing to look at your thoughts and beliefs objectively and commit to working with them.

2. Take out a piece of paper and list everything you can think of that is hard about T1D. Don't hold back!

3. After you finish writing, review everything on your list with a critical (and honest) eye. Circle the things that are legitimately hard about T1D.

4. Star the things you haven't been completely honest with yourself about. These may be challenging, but not as tough as you're making them out to be in your mind.

In the following chapters, we are going to take a closer look at the truth about T1D.

CHAPTER 2 KEY TAKEAWAYS

- *You have to be honest with yourself about the challenges of T1D.*

- *The first step is identifying what aspects of diabetes are difficult for you. The more specific you can be, the better.*

- *Naming your challenges is an uncomfortable but necessary step to handling T1D.*

- *It's easy to fall into the habit of not being honest with yourself. You're not dishonest on purpose; you're self-sabotaging.*

- *When you're not honest with yourself, you set yourself up for failure. When you're honest with yourself, you set yourself up for success.*

- *Honesty about the challenges of T1D is difficult but always worth it.*

Chapter 3

LET'S BE HONEST

HONESTY AND TRANSPARENCY MAKE YOU VULNERABLE. BE HONEST AND TRANSPARENT ANYWAY.

—MOTHER TERESA

WHAT IS IT about T1D that is so hard?

So many things!

I keep a running list of what people tell me makes T1D challenging for them. Here are some of the most common reasons I've heard over the past several years:

Feel free to put a check next to the reasons you identify with.

❑ High blood sugar ❑ Low blood sugar
❑ Constant decision-making ❑ Mental gymnastics
❑ Balancing act ❑ Difficult emotions
❑ Unpredictability ❑ Devices on your body
❑ All the stereotypes ❑ No breaks
❑ Everything you must carry ❑ Knowing it'll never go away
❑ The cost ❑ Feeling like a pincushion

- ❏ Interruptions to daily life
- ❏ Anxiety about lows
- ❏ Relationship with food
- ❏ Exhaustion
- ❏ Sleep
- ❏ Worry about complications
- ❏ Loss of control
- ❏ Inability to be spontaneous

We need to talk about some of the hard truths of T1D.

Living with type 1 diabetes isn't easy. Sometimes it can be downright daunting. As much as you may want to, there is no reason to pretend it's not. As we talked about in the last chapter, to handle T1D, you have to be honest with yourself about the challenges.

This chapter will focus on the reasons why T1D can be so difficult. My goal is to give you the facts about the stress of T1D and the challenges you may face in response to this stress.

There are a couple of things I hope you'll take away from reading this chapter.

First, I hope you'll recognize that your challenges are real. The things we're talking about in this chapter are experiences most people will have at some point in their life with diabetes. You're not alone in what you're experiencing, and you certainly aren't making these things up. When you accept that the challenges of T1D are not in your imagination, you can take steps to navigate these challenges with skill.

Pretending these hurdles aren't real or that they are not a big deal isn't helpful. Not only does this way of thinking prevent you from dealing with the issue at hand, but it also makes you feel guilty for feeling something you think you "shouldn't" be feeling.

Second, I want you to be able to identify what parts of T1D are the most difficult for you. In this chapter, we will talk about a wide range of emotional challenges people with T1D face.

Third, I want you to be able to give your challenges a name. Naming your experiences makes them real. They move from being vague and amorphous feelings to something you can think about and try to understand. When you name your diabetes-related challenges, they become easier to cope with. I know this may sound like backward logic, but I am going to ask you to trust me on this one.

The Most Challenging Part of T1D

Before we start talking about the reasons why T1D is difficult, I want to acknowledge that admitting diabetes is hard and you're having a hard time with it can be a scary step to take. But it's an important one.

Admitting to yourself that T1D is hard may be cathartic, but it's not easy. This process can be scary for a couple of reasons. Admitting T1D is difficult means acknowledging you have a chronic disease that likely will be with you for the rest of your life. I have met many people who think that if they pretend diabetes is easy, or worse, like it's not there, then it might somehow magically disappear. When you allow yourself to say that diabetes is challenging, you squash that dream—not that it was ever realistic in the first place.

Maybe even scarier is admitting you're having a hard time with T1D. If you're like most people, you like to think of yourself as strong, even invincible. Life with T1D changes this perception. People use words like different, weak, or broken to describe themselves when they have a tough time with T1D. Acknowledging you feel this way can seem like you're accepting defeat.

Remember, admitting you're having a hard time does nothing to change reality. The stress of T1D is still there whether or not you acknowledge it. Confronting what is truly going on can be scary, but acknowledging reality is the only way to change your experience with T1D.

Admitting you're having a hard time with T1D may not be easy, but it's always worth it.

T1D Is a Lot of Work

The day you were diagnosed with type 1 diabetes, your life changed forever. A new responsibility was handed to you. There will never be another day when you don't have to think about and manage your diabetes. And let's face it, managing T1D is a lot of work.

There is a common misconception by people who don't live with T1D, including many health care professionals, that diabetes is a check-the-box condition. From the outside, managing diabetes may look like a lot of work, but the tasks involved seem easy. If you check your blood sugar, take insulin, eat healthily, and get some exercise, you have checked all the boxes of diabetes management, and everything will work out just fine.

If only it were that simple—and we all know it's not.

Instead of checking a couple of boxes every day, managing T1D is like juggling while you're riding a unicycle on a busy street full of potholes in the middle of a hurricane. To stay on the unicycle, you have to constantly think about where you are now, where you're headed, and what the road and weather conditions will be like in a couple of hours. Then you have to be ready to change course at any time because of factors you haven't even thought of.

Managing T1D is exhausting. You constantly have to think, calculate, and look to the future. You're making hundreds of decisions a day to stay alive and healthy.

With all the time and brainpower put into managing diabetes, you would think you'd get a break every once in a while. Even the most demanding jobs allow for some time off. But T1D doesn't follow those rules. There are no days off. You are on nights, weekends, and holidays. Your diabetes requires constant care and feeding, which means the work of managing T1D is never-ending.

Exercise

Take a minute and make a list of everything you've done today to manage diabetes. Be sure to include:

- *All the tasks (for example, checking blood sugar, taking insulin, changing pump site)*

- *All the decisions you made (how much insulin to take, when to treat a low, whether or not it is safe to exercise, whether or not you needed to take action when you saw your blood sugar, etc.)*

- *All the calculations you made (e.g., counting carbs, correcting highs, how long the insulin in your pump/pen will last)*

- *All the preparation and planning for the rest of the day (what you need to take with you to manage your blood sugars, including glucose, insulin, backup pump supplies, etc.)*

Managing T1D is a lot of work. It means constantly paying attention to your blood sugars and making multiple decisions every day, with no breaks. All this work is exhausting, but that's not all. There are other reasons why T1D is challenging.

The Physical Toll of T1D

No matter how well you manage your blood sugars, there are going to be days where diabetes slows you down, or worse, knocks you to the ground. For people with T1D, there is no such thing as having perfect blood sugars all the time. You have diabetes, and out-of-range glucose levels come with the territory. Often, you can deal with a high or low, and it's not that big of a deal. But there are times when diabetes makes you feel awful. On those days, living with T1D is no easy feat.

When your blood sugar is very high (over about 250 mg/dl) you feel heavy, sluggish, and achy. When your blood sugar is very low (under about 50 mg/dl) you feel shaky, lightheaded, and weak. And when your blood sugar is on a roller coaster, going from high to low and back to high again, you feel like you've been hit by a bus. Sometimes, you don't recover quickly with these highs and lows, and you don't feel well for a while, even the rest of the day. These blood sugar swings can have a big impact on your life. When your blood sugar is out of range, you may have trouble focusing on your work. You may not want to be around other people. You may even just want to lie down and do nothing because you have no energy.

DR. MARK'S T1D

I've had many times in my life with T1D when my blood sugars have knocked me to the ground. One that always comes to mind is the time I was in Italy with my family. We were out on a day trip, and my blood sugar dropped dangerously low. We were out somewhere in the countryside, and I started feeling shaky and sweaty. I grabbed a soda I had brought with me and drank it, and not long after, my blood sugar came back up. My meter told me I was fine, but I felt like I'd been hit by a bus. I tried to push on but was having a tough time. I had a massive headache and felt exhausted. I ended up going back to our rental and staying in bed the rest of the day.

That day, the score was Diabetes 1 – Dr. Mark 0.

There is no doubt that T1D can take a physical toll every so often—and for some people, more than that. And when you don't feel well, T1D is hard. There may be days when the physical toll makes it hard to continue with your day.

Other times, the impact may not be so dramatic, but it's still there. The bottom line is that, even with the best management, there will be days when diabetes doesn't leave you feeling well.

The Emotional Toll of T1D

When you were first diagnosed, you probably spent time with your doctor and a Certified Diabetes Care and Education Specialist (CDCES) learning about managing T1D. You learned how to give yourself an injection, the difference between basal and rapid-acting (mealtime) insulin, and what to do when your blood sugar goes low. You probably felt scared, confused, and overwhelmed. You tried to make sense about what having T1D would mean for your life from that day forward, and you were trying to get steady on your feet managing your blood sugars.

I would be willing to bet that nobody said a word to you about the emotional challenges of T1D. For many people, the ongoing emotional struggles are a surprise, and we certainly don't talk about them enough.

The truth is, some of the most challenging aspects of living with T1D are emotional. Let's take a closer look at them.

Negative Emotions

If you live with T1D, I'm sure diabetes has brought up some negative emotions for you. Feelings such as frustration, anger, fear, guilt, shame, and many more are par for the course with T1D.

If T1D brings on any difficult emotions, I promise you're not crazy and you're not doing anything wrong. Your emotions are a natural reaction to the stress of living with diabetes. They signal to your brain that something isn't right, and they can push you to take action. T1D can be stressful at times, and, unfortunately, uncomfortable feelings are part of living with the condition.

There are many different things about T1D that can spur uncomfortable emotions. Sometimes it's something minor like hearing your CGM alarm or someone making an ignorant comment. It's the guilt you feel when you see your blood sugar skyrocket because you didn't pre-bolus or were impatient and overtreated a low. Then, of course, significant stressors like being hospitalized or being diagnosed with complications can bring on challenging feelings. Negative emotions about diabetes also can come out of nowhere and just be part of the ongoing stress of living with T1D.

REAL-LIFE T1D: THEO

Theo started his day in a bad mood. His CGM woke him up at least three times during the night. He was not only exhausted but also annoyed with himself. He ate pizza for dinner last night, knowing it would make his blood sugar rise, but he didn't take an extended bolus. Now he's frustrated, tired, and has a high blood sugar headache. These feelings are nothing new for Theo. He feels this way all the time.

These emotions about diabetes are having a negative impact on Theo's life. Recently, he was written up at work after snapping at his co-worker in front of a customer. The same day, Theo's girlfriend told him she's tired of him taking his frustrations about diabetes out on her. She warned that if they're going to continue their relationship, he needs to find a better way of dealing with his stress.

Theo realizes something needs to change. His problems at work and with his girlfriend were wake-up calls for how his negative feelings about diabetes affect his life. Even though he knows he needs to change something, he feels stuck in these feelings. Theo knows there will always be stressful parts of living with T1D. It just comes with the territory.

Negative Emotions about T1D in Real Life

The negative emotions that can come with T1D can affect your life in a lot of different ways. Not only are these emotions uncomfortable on their own, but they also can impact your daily life and the people around you. You have feelings, and then you react to them. Theo saw these challenges firsthand. His anger and frustration related to his blood sugars took a big toll on his self-esteem, making it harder to manage his diabetes. His feelings also crept into other areas of his life, causing him trouble at work and upsetting his girlfriend.

These negative emotions around T1D aren't fun. They can be uncomfortable, both mentally and physically. By their nature, difficult feelings can make you angry, depressed, or even hopeless. They make you feel out of control and give you a pessimistic outlook on T1D and other areas of your life. Feeling stressed or anxious can make you tense and drain your energy. So, it should be no surprise these emotions affect how you show up in the world.

When you're having a hard time with T1D, you might find that you lose your motivation to manage your diabetes. Or, like Theo, you may find yourself getting annoyed and angry at others or withdrawing from relationships that are important to you. When diabetes makes you angry or upset, it also can make it harder to focus on your work. And, of course, when T1D makes you feel frustrated, angry, and upset, you probably do what you can to try to forget about diabetes and how it makes you feel. No one wants to experience these negative emotions; they are no fun.

T1D-related Anxiety

It would be an understatement to say that anxiety is part of life with T1D. Research shows that the lifetime prevalence of generalized anxiety disorder in people with diabetes is just under 20%, or about 1 in 5 people. The numbers are even higher if we look at people who have anxiety about things that are specific to diabetes.

Anxiety is worry or fear about the future or something with an unknown outcome. If there is one thing that fills the minds of people with diabetes, it's worry and uncertainty. Anxiety has many faces for people with T1D. Let's take a closer look at a few of them.

First, there's the constant parade of thoughts about things that could happen in the short-term that get the mind racing and keep people up at night.

Did I take the right amount of insulin?

Will my blood sugar come down? How fast?

Will I have enough supplies with me on my trip?

What am I going to do if my pump breaks?

Can I handle it if my blood sugar goes low?

Do I have enough insulin to get me through the month?

The number of things to worry about sometimes feels like it can go on forever.

Diabetes also can cause social anxiety. It is common for people with diabetes to worry about what others will think about them because they have diabetes. Worrying that others will see them as sick, weak, or unattractive leads them to hide diabetes from the people in their life.

Anxiety also can extend to how people think about their health care team. Fear that a doctor will scold you because you're not managing diabetes perfectly (whatever that means) can make people hesitant to be completely open and honest with their health care team.

Worrying about developing complications is another cause of anxiety for people with diabetes, especially those who have difficulty managing their blood sugars. Complications are scary, and for some people, complications sit front and center in their thoughts about their future with diabetes.

REAL-LIFE T1D: AMBER
Since she was diagnosed with T1D three years ago,

going low has been on Amber's mind. She's terrified of low blood sugar, and her fear has crept into almost every part of her life. She under-boluses when she eats, sending her blood sugars high and making her tired and nauseous. Amber loves skiing and riding her bike, but she hasn't done either for three years because she's worried about going low. Her anxiety has paralyzed her and made her feel trapped.

Yesterday, Amber's roommate invited her to go out for happy hour. As much as she wanted to go, Amber told her roommate she was busy. The truth is, she declined because she was worried about what would happen if she went low at the restaurant. Amber's mind immediately raced to how embarrassed and helpless she would be if she had low blood sugar while they were out. At that moment, Amber realized how stuck her fear of hypoglycemia made her feel and how it's keeping her from doing things she wants to do.

T1D-related Anxiety in Real Life

People describe their anxiety around T1D in different ways.

Some people experience physical anxiety, describing it as a constant flow of electricity through their body. It is always there and is ready to zap them at any minute. This charge keeps them on their toes, aware of what is going to happen or what might happen next, always with a sense of nervousness.

Others describe their anxiety as something that makes their body jitter. They feel jumpy and like they're always on guard. This is what Amber experienced. The physical symptoms brought on by her intense worry made it hard for her to enjoy life because it felt like her anxiety was always there, front and center. Even if the mind is calm, the anxiety is still there in the body with feelings of restlessness, rapid breathing, heartbeat, sweating, fatigue, nausea, and even digestive issues.

Diabetes-related anxiety can show up mentally as well. Racing thoughts, constant worry about what might happen in the future, and overthinking situations are the most common symptoms of what some call "head anxiety." This type of anxiety can make it hard to do anything because you feel like you cannot think straight. It's easy to get lost in these anxious thoughts, preventing you from focusing on what you'd prefer to be thinking about.

Diabetes Burnout

It's no secret that managing T1D takes a lot of work. Diabetes burnout is when the tasks and emotional burden of managing T1D get to be too much. It's when you're sick and tired of having to think about T1D all the time, and you just want to give up and ignore diabetes for a while, or worse, forever.

Unfortunately, diabetes burnout is common, and most people with T1D experience it at some point. After all, living with T1D means having to be "on" 24/7, and as much as you'd like one, there are no breaks.

If you stop putting in the work to manage T1D because you feel burned out, it doesn't mean you don't want to be healthy or are lazy. It means the work of T1D feels overwhelming, and you're tired of the constant and seemingly never-ending grind.

REAL-LIFE T1D: TAYLOR

The first words out of Taylor's mouth when she walked into my office were, "I'm done with diabetes." She went on to tell me that she couldn't remember the last time she checked her blood sugar. Over the past three months, she had only taken insulin sporadically. Dealing with T1D, on top of her stressful job and taking care of her two young sons, had just gotten to be too much. Something had to give, and Taylor decided that thing was T1D.

Taylor felt like she was stuck between a rock and a hard place. She felt awful most of the time. At the same time, she had no motivation to take care of herself. After living with T1D for almost 15 years, she couldn't figure out how not to feel burned out. When she tried—and failed—to find motivation and get over these feelings, she ended up feeling even worse, both physically and emotionally.

Her burnout started bleeding into other areas of her life. For the past two years, Taylor has wanted to find a new job. She found several she was interested in but felt like she was in a rut when it came to taking the next step. Taylor already was having a tough time with diabetes, and she couldn't find the motivation to apply for a new job with T1D always on her mind. Taylor's burnout made her feel stuck in every part of her life, and she had no idea what to do.

Diabetes Burnout in Real Life

Diabetes burnout shows up in different ways for different people.

For Taylor, burnout meant doing everything she could to ignore T1D to avoid feeling so overwhelmed. Her frustration, combined with having a hard time getting motivated, made her feel like she was done with diabetes.

Even though diabetes burnout doesn't look the same for everyone, there are some common signs and symptoms. For example, people who feel burned out often have strong negative feelings about diabetes such as anger, frustration, guilt, and self-blame. Other people describe diabetes burnout as feeling like T1D is always in control of how they think and act, and there's nothing they can do about it. For others, burnout feels like they are isolated and alone with diabetes and have no one who "gets it" to support them.

Diabetes burnout and the feelings that come with it are not fun, but often, the more significant issue is how feeling burned out makes you behave. In an attempt to escape feeling burned out, people try to ignore diabetes. They figure that if they can get T1D out of their minds, they can finally get the break from it they've been dreaming about. Unfortunately, this strategy almost always backfires, leaving them even more stressed out and overwhelmed by diabetes.

Other Things that Make T1D Stressful

We can talk all day about the reasons why living with T1D is challenging. These include:

- *Relationships with friends and family*

- *Relationship with your health care team*

- *The logistics of managing T1D*

- *The financial burden of T1D*

- *The fact that sometimes T1D just makes no sense*

The bottom line is, T1D is challenging for many different reasons.

The Most Infuriating Thing about T1D

The struggle of living with T1D goes beyond all the work and how diabetes makes you feel. These things are problematic on their own. They don't feel good. They take up time and energy. They are exhausting, both physically and mentally.

But the most infuriating thing about T1D is how all these other challenges get in your way. When you're stressed—no matter where the stress is coming from—it's a lot more challenging to do the things that are important to you.

Constantly thinking about and preparing for what's next with T1D makes it harder to be present in your life with friends and family.

Feeling anxious about your blood sugars can make it difficult to sleep.

When you don't feel well because your blood sugar is out of range, you may have to cancel plans you were excited about.

Don't take it from me. Here's how some of my patients describe the ways diabetes gets in their way:

- *I get so anxious about going low when I'm asleep. I lay awake in bed for several hours, thinking about going low. Usually, I end up eating something, and I don't take insulin for it. My blood sugar goes high, and even though I can fall asleep because I'm not anxious, I wake up the next morning feeling like garbage.*

- *Traveling with diabetes takes too much preparation. I would love to travel, but I don't because all the work it takes to get ready just isn't worth it.*

- *I get so angry with my diabetes. No matter what I do, it feels like my blood sugars just don't cooperate. My anger bleeds into my relationships with my family, especially my fiancé. We've gotten in some blowout fights when I'm irritable because my blood sugar is high.*

- *Whenever my four-year-old daughter asks me to ride bikes with her, I always make up an excuse because I can't risk having low blood sugar while we're out.*

- *When my blood sugar goes high during a meeting at work, I have to leave. I don't feel well, and I have a hard time fully participating. I also don't want to worry about what my co-workers think about me when I get quiet and have to get up and go to the bathroom every fifteen minutes.*

All the uncomfortable thoughts, feelings, and emotions that come with diabetes make it challenging enough to live life the way you want. When diabetes makes it challenging to do what you want to do, you end up getting more upset and frustrated, adding to the burden even more.

You Think You Can't Handle the Challenges

The truth is T1D is hard, and there may not always be a way to make it easier.

What adds insult to injury is your belief that you cannot handle the challenges of T1D. Yes, T1D is stressful. But when you tell yourself you can't handle it, you trap yourself. You're in your way and you are stuck. If you think you can't handle the very real struggles of living with T1D, then those challenges weigh you down even more.

Believing you can handle the stress of T1D won't make it go away. But it does make it easier to deal with. You can approach the challenges of T1D with the confidence that you'll be able to figure out how to live the life you want, even with diabetes. And once you figure that out, you already are well on your way to handling T1D.

Honesty Helps You Cope

You cannot handle the challenges you don't acknowledge. Once you know what you are up against in your life with T1D, you can start facing your challenges head-on and learn the skills needed to handle them. Being honest with yourself and those you trust about T1D's hurdles is an essential first step to handling it.

Exercise

The following exercise will help you take an honest look at the challenges you face with T1D.

1. Brainstorm all the things about T1D that are challenging for you. Write down everything you can think of, even if you are not sure it's genuinely a challenge.

2. Look over your list and give each challenge a one-word name.

3. One by one, describe what each of these challenges feels like. Be sure to include the emotions, thoughts, physical feelings, and anything else you think is essential.

4. Describe how each challenge affects your daily life. How do they get in your way? Are there ways they help you?

5. After you finish this exercise, look over your list. What is it like to acknowledge the challenges of T1D in your life?

—————— CHAPTER 3 KEY TAKEAWAYS ——————

- *Life with T1D is challenging.*

- *Your challenges with T1D are real. They are not easy to deal with.*

- *It is crucial to identify and name your specific challenges. Vague is not helpful. Even though this may be uncomfortable to face, the more specific you can be about what you're experiencing, the better.*

- *The most stressful aspects of living with T1D include the work of T1D and emotions like anxiety and burnout.*

- *These challenges get even more stressful when they get in the way of doing things that are important to you.*

- *When you believe you cannot handle the stressful parts of T1D, you get stuck in these challenges and feel like you have no way out.*

Chapter 4

LET'S BE EVEN
MORE HONEST

YOU'RE GOING TO FIND THAT MANY
OF THE TRUTHS WE CLING TO DEPEND
GREATLY ON OUR OWN POINT OF VIEW.

—OBI-WAN KENOBI

HONESTY WORKS BOTH ways. In the last chapter, we talked
about all the reasons T1D is challenging. It sucks sometimes; there is no doubt about that.

But is it possible that sometimes you make diabetes out to
be more complicated than it really is?

For most people, the answer is yes.

The human brain tends to take something objectively
difficult, like type 1 diabetes, and turn it into something
even more complicated. When you do this with T1D, not
only are you not being honest with yourself, you also get
stuck in a place where diabetes is more challenging than
it needs to be.

If you're going to learn that you can handle T1D, you need to make sure what you're experiencing is truly stressful. Tough stuff that isn't truly tough, but that you've come to believe is tough, will be impossible to handle.

Let's take a closer look at some of the reasons why you make diabetes harder than it needs to be, and what you can do to be more honest with yourself about the realities of living with T1D.

You Make T1D Harder Than It Actually Is

Honesty goes beyond talking about the challenges of living with diabetes. It also means not letting yourself believe that diabetes is more stressful than it actually is.

You're probably not aware that you do this, but you do. We all do, to a certain degree. It is the way the human mind operates. We exaggerate things. We make them out to be more than they really are. This happens, but it's rarely helpful.

Nobody wants T1D to be challenging or stressful. I certainly don't, and I'm sure you don't either. But if diabetes is stressful, make sure there's a legitimate reason for your stress. Exaggerating the challenges of T1D is not fair to you.

We tend to let the stressful parts of T1D run away from us. The emotional burden of T1D gets bigger in our minds and more difficult to rein in. Stress that's based in reality is manageable because there's something tangible to focus on and deal with. For example, your blood sugar is high, your CGM alarm is going off in the middle of class, or your mom nags you nonstop about what you're eating. All these things are stressful for reasons you can identify.

On the other hand, sometimes you experience challenges around T1D that exist only in your thoughts. This stress isn't based in reality and turns into a runaway train. It becomes all-consuming. You try to deal with it, you try to contain it, but because it doesn't arise from something that you can identify, containing it becomes impossible. You get swallowed up in it, and there's nothing you can do. The pressure starts to take over your life.

REAL-LIFE T1D: HENRY

When his high alarm sounded for the third time that night, Henry got angry. He thought he took enough insulin for the ice cream sundae he ate earlier that evening, but apparently, he hadn't. Henry was sick and tired of feeling sick and tired of diabetes, especially in the middle of the night. As he lay in his bed, his thoughts ran away from him.

"I'm never going to be able to figure out this diabetes thing."

"T1D has shown me how stupid I really am."

"Nobody is ever going to want to be with me if I can't keep my blood sugars under control."

"I can't deal with all the stress T1D is throwing on me."

Eventually, Henry fell back asleep. When he woke up the following day, he still felt a wave of intense anger toward diabetes that he couldn't shake.

You can see how Henry took something that was objectively irritating and poured fuel on it so that it became much bigger than it needed to be. Nobody enjoys being woken up by their CGM multiple times in a night. That is annoying. But for Henry, the annoyance didn't end there. It took on a life of its own, which only served to make the situation much more complicated than it needed to be.

You Are Not Trying to Sabotage Yourself

When I say that you may make T1D more stressful than it needs to be, I am not blaming you here. While thinking this way isn't helpful, it doesn't mean you're doing anything wrong. And you're certainly not trying to sabotage yourself, at least not purposefully.

You Are Trying to Keep Yourself Safe

We all tend to exaggerate the challenging stuff in our lives. It's how we're wired, and it's one of the ways our minds try to keep us safe. Your brain thinks the stress you're feeling about diabetes serves a function. Your brain thinks it needs to keep you safe from the stress, so it makes it bigger than it is. The only problem is this way of thinking keeps you a little too safe because it keeps you stuck. You feel you can't handle the emotional challenges of T1D, so you don't even try.

You Are Trying to Find Answers

We all want T1D to make sense. I certainly do!

You want to know why your blood sugars are all over the place, even though you did everything "right."

You want to know why you are feeling burned out, frustrated, or out of control.

You want to know why you drew the short stick and got T1D in the first place.

These questions are all reasonable. Sometimes you may be able to find an answer, while other times, there is no answer, at least not one that makes sense. But you still want answers, even when there isn't an obvious one.

Your Stories About T1D

You make up stories to try to make sense of a confusing situation, and you hope these stories will help explain the unexplainable. But usually, all they do is make the problem seem worse than it already is. The stories you tell yourself are the unnecessary fuel for the T1D fire, and they make you believe that diabetes is much harder than it actually is.

Don't get me wrong. T1D sucks. But you need to be honest with yourself about how much it sucks and rein in your stories when they aren't based in fact.

Your stories about T1D almost always have some grain of truth to them. Something happens in your life with T1D that, by all objective measures, sucks. Maybe your blood sugar goes high for no good reason. Maybe your pump tubing gets caught on a doorknob. Or maybe someone makes an ignorant comment about diabetes that makes you feel self-conscious. There are countless things about T1D that suck—and nobody would argue that these things don't suck.

But then, these objectively stressful situations quickly take on a life of their own. You try to make sense of why this challenging situation happened. You want an explanation but can't find one. So you make one up. And from there, your story, and your stress, take off.

The stories you tell yourself about T1D all follow a similar pattern. As you work to be more honest with yourself about diabetes, notice the stories you're telling and ask yourself whether they're based in fact.

The Anatomy of a Story

To figure out whether your stories are based in fact, you have to understand the anatomy of them. When you know how these stories develop in your mind, you'll have an easier time assessing them. If you find they're not based in fact, you can stop them in their tracks.

Your stories about T1D form in four steps:

- **Trigger:** *Something happens in your life with T1D.*

- **Meaning-making:** *You come up with an explanation for why this thing happened.*

- **Time travel:** *With the meaning you gave the story, you start thinking about what you should have done differently in the past or what you have to do in the future to make things better.*

- **Blowback:** *You do whatever you can think of to try to control the discomfort that comes from the story, which only makes things worse.*

Let's take a closer look at each of the four steps of the anatomy of your stories about T1D.

Step #1: Trigger

The unexpected and the frustrating happen with T1D all the time. I sometimes describe living with T1D as playing a never-ending game of dodgeball. You are constantly trying to figure out how to avoid getting tagged by a ball. But no matter what you do, you're going to get hit. It's just the nature of the game. The only difference is T1D is not a game.

These triggers are situations that actually took place in your life with T1D, and they suck. The number of triggers with T1D is endless. Here are some examples:

- *Your blood sugar goes high.*

- *You want to go to sleep, but you can't because you're low.*

- *Your CGM alarm goes off in the middle of an important work meeting.*

- *Someone makes an ignorant comment about T1D.*

- *Your pump site rips out, and you have to make everyone wait while you change it.*

This list is by no means complete; there is an infinite number of trigger events that can take place. Triggers are simply the things that make T1D challenging. And there are many.

In the anatomy of a story, triggers are not a problem. Triggers are expected. It's what happens after the trigger that can cause challenges.

Step #2: Meaning-making

When trigger events happen, they can make you feel out of control and even helpless. These feelings are not fun. Naturally, you're going to want to try to understand why these occur. If you know why they took place, you can take action to make sure they don't happen again.

There will be times when there is an obvious reason why the trigger took place. Understanding why something happened makes you feel like you have some level of control, and who doesn't want to feel like they have some control over diabetes? But as you know, T1D does not always make sense. This means there will be plenty of times when you just cannot figure out why the stress is there.

When the reason is a mystery, we tend to do whatever we can to find an answer. And when we can't come up with an explanation, we do the next obvious thing. We make one up, even when this explanation has a shaky basis in truth.

Meaning-making is coming up with an explanation for why something happened in your life with T1D or why diabetes makes you feel a certain way. When there is no other explanation for what happened, you fall back on what you know—yourself.

Meaning-making is the story you tell yourself to solve the mystery of why something occurred. But it goes deeper than just why this situation came up. Our stories usually go beyond the facts of the situation. They dive into what we think having diabetes means about us. The meaning you make is rarely based in fact, at least not entirely. And you usually cast yourself as the villain in the story.

Here are some examples of stories you might tell yourself as you try to make sense of why something happened in your life with T1D:

- *Diabetes makes me weak and broken.*

- *I am a failure, and I'll never get this blood sugar thing right.*

- *Diabetes will always be hard for me.*

- *My CGM and pump make me unattractive.*

- *I'm always going to be anxious when my blood sugar is low.*

- *I can't handle all this stress around diabetes.*

- *Having diabetes means I can't...*

Exercise

Do any of the stories above sound familiar to you? Take a minute and make a list of the stories you tell yourself about what having T1D means about you, what you can and cannot do, and about the future. You may not be able to identify all your stories right now, and that's okay. Keep a running list. The more you notice your stories, the more you will be aware of them when they come up.

Your stories about T1D make things challenging enough on their own. However, they usually do not stop there. Once a story forms, it starts to take on a life of its own.

Step #3: Time Travel

Think back to the last time you got lost in a great book. You were so immersed in the story that everything around you became a blur. Transported to another time and place in your mind, you were unaware of what was happening around you. Kids playing, people talking, your phone ringing—none of these distractions could bring you back.

Your stories about what having T1D means about you work in the same way. It's easy to get lost in these stories. They take you out of the present moment and get you thinking about what you should have done differently in the past and what the future holds.

There is a difference between your stories about T1D and the ones you get lost in while reading a book on the beach. Your stories about what diabetes means about you and your future are not stories that you want to be immersed in. They are not exciting, and they certainly are not helpful. To be emotionally healthy with T1D, you have to be honest with yourself about the realities of diabetes. When your stories about T1D take you away from reality, that's usually a good sign the story is not based in fact and that you're not being completely honest.

Your stories make things worse. Time-travel with your T1D stories is like adding fuel to a fire that already may be burning out of control. And there is nothing you can do about it. You can only change how you relate to T1D right here, right now. Change is not possible when your mind is lost in the past or the future.

Step #4: Blowback

Getting lost in your stories about T1D isn't fun. You ruminate about things you should have done in the past or things that might happen in the future. These stories take place in your mind, but they affect your real life. This impact shows up in your behavior.

Your stories about T1D and what it means about you do not make you feel good about yourself. They are uncomfortable, and like any normal human, you try to control uncomfortable feelings. The downside is this strategy almost always comes back to bite you.

Blowback is how you act when these stories are swirling around in your head. These are the stories that cause you to stay home and avoid activities. They make you lash out at other people. Blowback from your stories may even cause you to slack off on taking care of your diabetes.

Think of a time when your stories about living with T1D drove your behavior. Maybe you heard your CGM high alarm go off for the fifth time that day, and you ripped off your sensor. Or perhaps a co-worker made a snarky comment when you pulled out your insulin pen to bolus for lunch and, embarrassed, you sank in your chair. Or maybe you yelled at your wife when she asked if you needed help treating a low.

All of these reactions come from a story you tell yourself about T1D, and none of them do anything to help you change your diabetes for the better. Your response to these stories almost always makes the situation worse. The blowback from your stories gives you short-term relief from an ongoing problem. At its root, the problem is not being honest with yourself about how much T1D sucks.

T1D does suck, but the way you think about it and the stories you tell yourself can make it suck a lot more than it actually does.

The Anatomy of Stories in the Real World

Let's deconstruct some stories people with T1D tell themselves.

Monica

- **Trigger:** *Monica's CGM reads 326 mg/dl.*

- **Meaning-making:** *Monica tells herself, "I'm a failure. This reading means I am never going to get this diabetes thing right."*

- **Time travel:** *Monica gets lost in her head, beating herself up over what she ate for lunch.*

- **Blowback:** *Monica rips off her CGM and doesn't check her blood sugar for the rest of the day.*

Tim

- **Trigger:** *Tim's doctor suggests he try using an insulin pump.*

- **Meaning-making:** *Tim tells himself that wearing an insulin pump means he has to accept he has a chronic condition.*

- **Time travel:** *When he thinks about wearing a pump, Tim gets consumed with thoughts about how much he hates T1D and how he doesn't want to deal with it.*

- **Blowback:** *Tim refuses even to give the pump a trial run.*

Jordan

- **Trigger:** *Jordan is on a first date. She orders food and drinks, and she knows she needs to take insulin.*

- **Meaning-making:** *Jordan tells herself, "I really like this guy, and if he finds out I have diabetes, he won't like me anymore."*

- **Time travel:** *Instead of focusing on her date, Jordan is trying to figure out how she can take insulin without him knowing.*

- **Blowback:** *Jordan leaves her date alone at the table for five minutes while she takes her insulin, leaving him feeling confused and a little bit suspicious.*

Your Stories Keep You Stuck

Your mind makes T1D harder than it needs to be, and this is not at all helpful. This approach to diabetes is problematic for several reasons, beyond the fact that you are not being honest with yourself, and the stories you are telling yourself are not accurate.

Not being honest with yourself and making T1D harder than it needs to be makes life difficult. This way of thinking gets in your way and keeps you stuck. My guess is this is the exact opposite of what you want to do.

Here is what happens when you are not honest with yourself and make life with T1D more complicated than it is.

Telling Yourself T1D Is Hard Makes It Hard

Instead of navigating life with T1D nimbly and with flexibility, it starts to feel like you're walking through mud. You thought diabetes got in your way before. With all those stories and meaning you pile on top, it starts to feel like even more of a burden. You stop living your life because T1D feels like it is too much to handle.

Maybe your stories tell you diabetes is dangerous, and you are weak. This combination is toxic. If diabetes is truly dangerous and you're weak, it makes perfect sense to withdraw and be more cautious. But neither of these statements is objectively true. Diabetes may feel dangerous, and you may feel weak, but feelings do not equal fact. But even so, your feelings keep getting in your way, in large part because your stories run rampant and unchecked.

The stories you tell yourself about diabetes and what it means about you make it more challenging to live your life on your terms. This makes you even angrier, which only gets you more stuck. And then you take more steps to stop living your life because it feels like even more of a hassle. You just want the stress to go away, and the only way you know to do this is to avoid and withdraw. The stories you tell yourself about diabetes can end up setting off a cascading effect of withdrawal from the things you want to spend your time doing.

Talk about a no-win situation!

But then things get even more challenging. When you avoid the emotional burden of T1D, it leads to more problems because you never allow yourself to discover the truth about your stories. Your stories tell you that you cannot handle T1D, and when you avoid stressful situations, you never get the chance to show yourself that you can handle diabetes. Instead, you use your avoidance behavior as evidence that you cannot handle the stress.

This way of thinking is built on faulty logic.

I'd be willing to bet big that you can handle T1D. But if you're stuck in your stories and are not willing to try to handle it, you'll never know for sure. Your stories about T1D paralyze you and become self-fulfilling. You believe you can't handle the tricky parts of diabetes, so you never try, which reinforces your belief that you cannot handle it, even though in reality, you can.

See how quickly this got really confusing?

REAL-LIFE T1D: STEPHANIE

Stephanie thought she had to plan a week ahead of time to go to the pool in her apartment building. She had to make sure her CGM and pump site were in places they wouldn't be visible to anyone in the vicinity. The mental gymnastics Stephanie played made going to the pool a big event in her week when it should have been a spur-of-the-moment decision. Stephanie was terrified of what people would think about her if they found out she had "robot" parts (her words). Even thinking of going to the pool set off what she would later call the "story machine" in her head.

"These devices make me ugly."

"Nobody will want to talk to me because I wear a pump."

"Diabetes devices and bathing suits cannot go together."

On the rare occasion when Stephanie's desire to go to the pool won out, she would plan out her pool visit with precision, getting lost in her head for hours working out the details and worrying about it. And then, when Stephanie finally made it to the pool, she always sat on the lounge in the corner away from everybody, never venturing anywhere close to the water.

With a lot of work, Stephanie was able to see that she was taking the simple act of going for a swim and making it a huge deal, and for no good reason. She paid the price for worrying about showing off her diabetes devices because it took up so much of her energy and made her time at the pool full of anxiety and self-consciousness.

Honesty Is Still the Best Policy with T1D

The bottom line is you need to be honest with yourself about how much T1D sucks. But you also need to be honest about how, sometimes, you make T1D much harder than it needs to be. It's all too easy to let T1D suck more than it needs to.

We get lost in our stories at times, and this way of thinking about T1D is not helpful for any of us. Honesty is always the best policy with T1D, especially when not being truthful about it makes diabetes more challenging than it has to be.

─────── **CHAPTER 4 KEY TAKEAWAYS** ───────

- *Honesty works both ways.*

- *We tend to take things about T1D that are objectively hard and make them a lot harder than they need to be.*

- *Life with T1D is confusing, and sometimes it doesn't make sense.*

- *You want T1D to make sense, and so you make up stories to help explain what's happening and why.*

- *You are not trying to sabotage yourself with your stories, even though they make T1D more challenging for you.*

- *The best way not to let your stories run away from you is to identify them, so you can stop them before they get out of control.*

Chapter 5

CONTROL IS NOT (ALWAYS) THE ANSWER

YOU CAN'T CONTROL HOW YOU FEEL, BUT YOU CAN ALWAYS CHOOSE HOW YOU ACT.

—MEL ROBBINS

CONTROL IS A funny thing. Sometimes when you try to get the upper hand on your experience with T1D, you end up feeling even more out of control.

My guess is you like to be in control. You'll go to great extremes to gain control in different areas of your life, especially with T1D.

You want to be in control of your blood sugars. You want to control your stress around diabetes. You want to control how other people treat you. You think if you can find ways to control these aspects of your life with T1D, it will reduce your anxiety and help you feel more stable on your feet.

You have probably tried some creative strategies to shape your experience with diabetes. You may not even be aware that what you're doing is an attempt to control different aspects of your life with T1D, and you do them without thinking about it. But in the end, there are some things about T1D you cannot rein in. And as much as you try to control your experience with diabetes, you never quite get there. You may think you'll be able to dictate how it looks, but in the end, this belief is an illusion.

What does this illusion of control look like for people with type 1 diabetes? Here are just a few examples:

- *You pretend you don't have diabetes.*

- *You get angry with T1D and have a hard time letting go of the anger.*

- *You don't check your blood sugar or take insulin in front of other people.*

- *You are glued to your CGM.*

- *You ignore your CGM alarms.*

- *You lie in bed trying to figure out how to make T1D suck less.*

- *You drink and/or smoke weed when diabetes gets overwhelming.*

- *You get sucked down rabbit holes on T1D-related social media.*

- *You plan where you will wear your diabetes devices so no one will see them.*

- *You spend a lot of time worrying about what others think about your diabetes.*

As hard as you try, these strategies to control your stress around T1D simply do not work.

Do they give you short-term relief? *Maybe.*

Do they control your stress in the long term? *No!*

Do they backfire and make T1D suck more than it already does? *Absolutely!*

What would it be like if you stopped trying to control the things about T1D that you have no control over? You know, your thoughts, emotions, how other people treat you. You can't always control your feelings of being overwhelmed, anxious, burned out, or frustrated. You can influence your blood sugars and your emotions, but you certainly cannot control them completely—and the more you try, the more you see that it's impossible. The irony is, the more you try to control these things, the more challenging they are to handle.

To cope with your uncomfortable emotions, you have to let go of the illusion you can control the parts of diabetes that suck. Letting go of control is a tall order.

REAL-LIFE T1D: SAM

Sam's diagnosis with T1D when he was 55 came out of the blue. Sam is athletic and takes pride in his health. He runs a successful landscaping business, and before he was told he had T1D, he was never sick a day in his life. Now seven years, later, Sam is on a quest for answers. For a couple of years after his diagnosis, he had convinced himself the doctors had made a mistake. The reality that he had T1D was too much to handle, so he pretended he was healthy. This strategy landed him in the hospital with diabetic ketoacidosis (DKA) four times. He finally has accepted that he has T1D, but now he is trying to find a cure. He has spent hours on the internet researching remedies and tens of thousands of dollars on doctors and supplements. Sam is exhausted, frustrated, and broke, but determined to keep searching for answers. The alternative, accepting he has to live with T1D for the rest of his life, is too much for him to handle.

Why You Grasp for Control

The day you were diagnosed with T1D, you probably felt entirely out of control. You had no idea what the future would hold. Your whole world had changed in an instant, and the life you had known up until that point felt like it was over. When you started learning how to manage T1D, hopefully, your blood sugars came back in range (at least some of the time). But you were still on edge. If diabetes could come out of the blue and rock your world, you started to wonder what could be next.

Then came everyday life with diabetes. You never knew what to expect. Some days your blood sugars were just fine, and other days they made absolutely no sense. Burnout, anxiety, and feeling overwhelmed started to occur with no rhyme or reason. You felt like you had no control over any aspect of your life with T1D, and in some ways, you were not too far off-base.

But you yearn for control. You want to feel stable. You want to feel confident that everything is going to be all right. You don't want to feel what you're feeling. You want to control your blood sugars, your emotions, and how you see yourself. If only you could figure out how to do this. You're convinced there is an answer out there, and all you have to do is find it.

So, you start looking for ways to control your experience, especially over the emotional aspect of T1D. You don't like how T1D makes you feel about yourself, and you want to change it. And the only way you know how to change the way T1D makes you feel is to try and control it, right?

But there's a problem. You haven't found the answer, at least not yet. Looking for control and not finding it is not only aggravating, it makes you feel even more out of control. The more out of control you feel, the harder you try to gain control, and the cycle continues.

You Want Answers

You think that to control the things about T1D you don't like, you have to understand why they're happening. Your blood sugar is high, so you try to figure out the reason. You're having trouble falling asleep because you're worried about going low in the middle of the night, so you want to figure out where your anxiety is coming from. You were feeling fine yesterday, and today you're feeling overwhelmed with the burden of T1D. You wonder what caused this sudden change.

You're convinced that if you can figure out why these things are happening, you can stop them. You're willing to go to great lengths to try and find the answers, even if it means not being completely honest with yourself.

You have decided there has to be a reason T1D makes you feel a certain way. The answer has to be either external or internal.

External Answers

An external explanation is something that happens outside of you. For example, if one of your co-workers makes a snide comment about your insulin pump or something you're eating, you can link your feelings to that person's comment. Or, if you have a big project due at work next week and you're stressed out, then you can reasonably assume your stress is causing your blood sugar to go high. While the explanation may not always be obvious, when you're able to figure out why something is happening, the next steps are pretty cut and dried. You know why your blood sugar is behaving in a certain way or why you're feeling the way you do, and it can be pretty easy to come up with a solution to fix it.

Maybe you avoid your co-worker or talk to the human resources department at your company about what your co-worker said and how it made you feel. If you know your blood sugar is high because of stress, either you find a way to reduce your stress, or you remember that this stressful time will not last for very long, and more than likely, your blood sugars will come down once it is over. In both of these examples, you found a reasonable external explanation for what you're experiencing with T1D.

Internal Answers

I've had type 1 diabetes for over 20 years. This means there has not been one day in over two decades that I have not taken insulin. But every once in a while, I will sit down to eat and forget to take insulin for my food. This happens more often than I like to admit, and I'm sure it happens to you sometimes as well.

When I forget to bolus for food, without fail, my blood sugar shoots up, and I know exactly why it happened. It's my fault. I forgot to do what I was supposed to do, and high blood sugar and frustration are never far behind. I can count many times when things I did or did not do affected my blood sugars and my emotions. I'm sure you can too. I am always learning from these situations and constantly working to improve. The explanation falls clearly in my lap. I can see what happened, and even though I don't like what I learn, I can see why it occurred.

But what happens when there isn't a clear explanation? What happens when you try and try, but you can't figure out a reason why T1D is making you feel overwhelmed or anxious? What happens when your blood sugar is not cooperating, and you can't understand why?

You want an answer, and there isn't an obvious one. Where do you look?

Most of the time, our go-to strategy is to look inward for an answer. If something is going wrong in my life with diabetes, and I can't figure out why, it must be my fault. It must be something I did. Or even worse, I am feeling this way because of a character defect caused by diabetes.

For example…

- *I did something to cause this.*

- *Diabetes makes me weak, so, of course, I am burned out.*

- *I am different because I have diabetes, so I'm embarrassed.*

- *I should have known the carb count on that menu was not accurate.*

- *If only I had done an extended bolus, I wouldn't have gone low.*

- *I'm not strong enough to keep diabetes from making me feel depleted.*

- *I can't handle all the stress of diabetes, so, of course, I am going to feel this way.*

- *Diabetes is too complicated, and I'm not smart enough to figure it out.*

Blaming yourself when you cannot come up with any other explanation for why you're having a tough time with T1D is something we all do. But placing the blame where it doesn't belong is not only unhelpful, it's dishonest.

What if there is no answer to why diabetes makes you feel a certain way or why your blood sugar is out of range? Or what if the only explanation is you have T1D, and there is nothing you can do about having diabetes?

I know that isn't the answer you want. Having no good answer means there's nothing you can do to change how you're feeling. With no answer, and no prospect of things getting any better, you even may be feeling hopeless. You're probably feeling like diabetes sucks, and there's no way you're ever going to be able to handle it.

I want to let you in on a secret.

The next thing you can do to handle the fact that diabetes sucks is to stop trying to find an answer to questions that don't have any. The best way to handle the challenging emotions that come with living with T1D is to stop trying to control them. Often with T1D, your attempt to control your experience is part of the problem, not the solution. Letting go of your attempt at control is the only way you can work to start handling the fact that T1D sucks. The more you try to control your experience, the more stuck you get in the reality that your experience with T1D sucks. Learning to handle T1D means getting unstuck, and getting unstuck sometimes means letting go of control.

Searching for answers to questions where no good answers exist and trying to control things that can't be controlled almost always makes things worse. You end up spending a lot of time and energy fighting battles you have no hope of winning. The resulting frustration ends up being even more stressful than the original experience you were trying to avoid. The effort you put into fighting this battle takes up a ton of headspace that you don't have.

Coming to a place of honesty with yourself and accepting that there may not be a way to control the challenging parts of diabetes isn't easy. It means you have to stop running away from the uncomfortable parts of T1D. It means you have to stop spending your energy fighting for control and searching for answers. It means accepting diabetes for what it is and accepting that sometimes T1D sucks.

But there is good news. When you stop searching for answers and accept that there are things about diabetes you cannot control, life with T1D usually becomes more manageable. You stop focusing on what you're trying to control and instead start focusing on the rest of your life. The challenging emotions are still there, but they become much less of a big deal.

Up to this point, you've been trying to control your experience with T1D, and it's not working. More likely than not, your current strategy will never work. Moving forward, you have a couple of options when you are confronted with the uncomfortable parts of T1D you can't control. The choice is yours, but my guess is you know that you can't keep doing what you're doing.

Here are your options:

- **Keep trying to control T1D:** *You've been trying this for a while now, without success. Just when you think you've found the answer, you realize* *it's not going to work. I know you want to keep trying to control your emotions around T1D, but this book is about honesty, so let's be truthful. What are the chances you'll be able to figure out how to control how diabetes makes you feel? Many people have tried (including me), but I don't know one person who has been successful in the long run (I certainly haven't). If you want to take this option, be my guest. But do it at your own risk. And remember that you can always change your mind if you choose this option and it doesn't work out.*

- **Accept T1D, but allow it to eat you up:** *Your head knows that you cannot control the stress of diabetes, but your heart isn't there. With this option, you have accepted you cannot control every part of your life with diabetes, but you're not ready to lean into the discomfort. The tension between what you know you have to do to be in a good place with diabetes and what you're willing to do to get there gets intense to the point that the discomfort of living with T1D eats you up.*

- **Handle it:** *You know that T1D sucks, and you also know the best option is to learn to deal with the fact that it sucks. You have realized that as much as you want to, trying to control the stress of diabetes only makes it worse. Leaning in may not be your first choice, but you know it's your best, and really the only, choice that will put you in a place where T1D will not get in your way. When you choose this option, you've concluded that even* *though you have T1D, you are strong, and, with the right set of skills, you'll be able to handle the stress, even when it seems complicated. You're confident that once you get to a place where you can handle T1D, it becomes a lot easier to deal with, and even though the emotional burden doesn't ever go away, it becomes a lot less of an issue.*

Letting Go of Control Is Not Easy

Accepting that T1D is challenging is not easy. It means letting go of control, and letting go of control is never easy. Be patient with yourself because coming to a place of acceptance doesn't happen overnight. If you're struggling with acceptance, cut yourself some slack and know this struggle is normal.

Be careful not to attach a story to the fact you're having a hard time accepting T1D. Your mind may go there and tell you stories such as...

- *The fact I'm having a hard time accepting T1D means it's better to keep fighting to control my feelings.*

- *Accepting T1D means giving in, and I refuse to give in.*

- *Diabetes has broken me down so much that acceptance is out of reach.*

- *Other people may be able to accept diabetes, but they are stronger than me. That's not something I'll ever be able to do.*

Attaching to these stories just puts another barrier in your path to acceptance. And acceptance is the only way you will handle T1D and move forward in your life.

Quick note ————————————————————————

Just because you can't control everything about T1D doesn't mean you have to throw your hands up in the air and surrender. There are aspects of your diabetes you can control, or at the very least, influence. In the following chapters, I'll give you some helpful tips for managing diabetes and teach you the skills you need to handle the stress when T1D gets challenging.

Ready to get started?

—————— **CHAPTER 5 KEY TAKEAWAYS** ——————

- *Humans like to feel in control, and living with T1D can make you feel out of control.*

- *People do lots of creative things to attempt to control their experience with T1D. These attempts are rarely successful.*

- *One thing people do while trying to gain control is look for explanations for why things are happening (e.g., why their blood sugar is high, why they feel burned out, etc.).*

- *Sometimes there is no good answer for why things happen with T1D.*

- *Looking for answers where none exist can make it harder to handle the stress of T1D.*

- *Work to get a handle on the things about T1D you can control (e.g., what you eat, how much insulin you take, when you exercise), let go of things you cannot control, and be mindful of the difference between these two categories.*

Chapter 6

YOU HAVE TO PUT IN THE WORK

YOU CAN'T HANDLE WHAT YOU DON'T MANAGE.

—DR. MARK

I REMEMBER THE first patient I saw who had T1D. A young college student, he had to leave school after the first semester of his freshman year after being hospitalized for DKA twice in as many months. His mom called and told me his story and asked if I would see her son. I had been thinking about focusing my practice on people with T1D, and this seemed like a great case to start with.

How hard could it be to help this young man understand how important it is to take care of his diabetes? When I hung up with his mom, I had what I thought was a brilliant treatment plan ready to go. All I would have to do is help him understand why high blood sugars are so dangerous. As a bonus, I would show him how managing his blood sugars and staying out of the hospital would help him feel better and live his best life as a college student.

Sounds simple, right?

Little did I know working with this young man would prove to be a lot more challenging than I initially had thought. At first, it seemed obvious to me that avoiding managing T1D was not a great solution.

The more I worked with this young man, the more I realized the real reasons he was not managing his diabetes were a lot more complicated. He wasn't lazy. It's not that he didn't understand the mechanics of managing his blood sugar. What he was doing (or not doing) was a symptom of something bigger. Ignoring diabetes at school was a symptom of his belief that he couldn't handle the stress of T1D.

More specifically, he thought he couldn't handle:

- *Feeling different.*

- *Feeling overwhelmed and burned out.*

- *The embarrassment of T1D.*

- *Figuring out how to enjoy college and manage T1D.*

- *Explaining T1D to the women he dated.*

The strategy he used to cope with his symptoms was only making it worse. Like scratching a bug bite, it helped him feel better in the moment but ended up making it more difficult for him to deal with his diabetes in the long run. He got comfortable not managing T1D, which only made it harder to handle. Ignoring T1D led to him leaving school and losing everything he was trying so desperately to keep.

I soon realized that even though ignoring diabetes was extreme, his strategy is not all that uncommon.

Have you ever tried to handle diabetes by ignoring it? Have you ever thought that the best way to cope with the stress is to slack off with your T1D management? Maybe you didn't stop managing diabetes altogether. Maybe you just cut corners here and there. You only checked your blood sugar when you felt it was out of range. You didn't bolus for snacks between meals. Maybe you took insulin without counting the carbs you were eating and just hoped for the best.

How did this strategy work? Did it help you handle diabetes better, or did it backfire and make life with T1D even more challenging in the long run?

Avoiding Managing T1D Is Not the Solution

I know it sounds obvious, but you must work to manage your diabetes.

You want to be able to live your life without letting diabetes get in your way. You want to be able to handle diabetes and deal with the challenges. When you avoid managing diabetes, it takes you in the exact opposite direction of your goal.

One of the most critical steps to handling T1D is to lean into the work of managing it. Your pancreas does not produce insulin. To stay alive, you have to take insulin. To keep your blood sugars down so you feel good and can function, you have to monitor your blood sugar, count carbs, and a whole lot more. No amount of wishful thinking is going to change this reality. It is impossible to take diabetes out of your life, and ignoring diabetes or pretending like you don't have it only makes the challenging parts an even bigger part of your life.

When you avoid the work of T1D, the emotional burden increases. You feel awful. It slows you down and makes the things you want to do a lot more complicated.

Have you ever tried not to think about something? How successful were you? Actively avoiding thinking about something that's always with you, like T1D, is a lot harder than it sounds. If you don't believe me, try it right now.

Look around and find something you can look at. It doesn't matter what it is—a clock, a plant, a chair, another person.

Once you have chosen that thing, don't think about it.

You can think about anything you want, but don't think about that one thing whatever you do.

Okay, how did you do? Were you able to avoid thinking about it?

I would be willing to bet you weren't very successful. How do I know? Because it is nearly impossible not to think about something you're trying to avoid. To avoid it, you have to think about it. You have to think about not thinking about it.

It's no different when you try to avoid thinking about T1D. You can choose not to manage diabetes, but choosing not to take care of it makes you think about it even more. You don't feel well, so the dark side of T1D is ever-present. But you also have to work to push diabetes aside in your mind.

You eat, and you know you need to take insulin but choose not to. You have to think about T1D to make that choice.

You can tell your blood sugar is high because you have been peeing every fifteen minutes all day, but you don't want to know your blood sugar reading. You have to think about diabetes and decide not to check your glucose.

You have two scoops of ice cream and don't want to think about how many carbs you ate, so you don't look at the nutrition facts and just give yourself 10 units of insulin, hoping you guessed correctly. That decision took thought, and now you'll be thinking about your blood sugar even more over the next couple of hours because you have no idea what it's going to do.

Another reason why avoiding diabetes makes it difficult to handle is because you're not on solid ground with your blood sugars. You avoid the work of diabetes because you want to feel stable and in control, and you think the only way this is possible is by moving diabetes out of the way. You soon find that avoiding managing T1D just makes you feel more unstable, making it more challenging to handle rather than less.

Wishing T1D will magically go away if you avoid thinking about it sounds like a dream, but it doesn't work and almost always turns into a nightmare.

There are two aspects of managing T1D that I want to focus on in this chapter. Both are essential steps to helping you handle the stress of diabetes. The first step is to understand what T1D is and the best way to manage it, taking your lifestyle into account.

You Can't Handle What You Don't Grasp

Imagine you have a big presentation to give at work. You've known about this presentation for weeks. The pressure is building in your mind, and a lot is riding on the decision that will come from what you say. You know you have to do prep work to understand what you're talking about to hit it out of the park. You can talk about the topic from a high level, but you're not familiar with it enough to discuss it in detail. Thinking ahead to the questions your client probably will ask terrifies you. Usually, you can get by with B.S. answers, but probably not this time. But you push off preparing for the presentation, partly because the details of the topic feel overwhelming and partly because you know that even with all the time in the world to prepare, there are still some aspects you'll never grasp entirely.

The meeting is getting closer and closer, and you don't do anything to get ready for it. In fact, you do whatever you can to avoid thinking about the meeting. As the date approaches, the more nervous you get. The information you need to rock this presentation is on your desk, but you ignore it.

The day of the meeting arrives, and you're terrified. You have no idea what you're going to say. You feel unprepared (because you are) and you're convinced the whole thing is going to be a bust, so you decide to call in sick.

Do you ever feel this way about diabetes? You know you need to lean in to really understand T1D, but instead, you turn away. You don't do the one thing that will help you get your sea legs with T1D. Instead, you stay stuck in your instability. Yet, you're still struggling to handle the stress of T1D.

If you're ever going to be able to handle T1D, something has to give. You're going to have to put in the work to understand your diabetes. You may be wondering what this work looks like. Here are steps you can take to help you grasp what affects your blood sugar.

Step #1: Lean into Your Data

Diabetes is a data-driven condition, and you can learn a lot from looking at and leaning into your numbers. If you're using a CGM, that's a great place to start. With blood sugar readings every five minutes, you can identify patterns in your blood sugars and make adjustments accordingly. You also can see how different foods, activities, and situations impact your blood sugar.

I know the prospect of leaning into your data may feel overwhelming. You may be scared not only of all the numbers but also of what you might find in your data. You may think that ignorance about your diabetes data is bliss, and you don't have to change what you don't know. But ignoring your data leaves you clueless about how to manage your blood sugars and erodes any hope of ever being confident in managing T1D. Simply put, ignoring your data makes T1D a lot tougher to handle.

Step #2: Use Your Resources

No one expects you to understand T1D on your own. Diabetes is complex, and you're going to need support as you get steady on your feet. An essential part of understanding diabetes is knowing where to turn when you need help. There is no shortage of resources available to support you in mastering the art of diabetes management. These resources include your endocrinologist and diabetes educator, others with type 1 diabetes, websites, blogs, podcasts, social media, and many more.

Step #3: Admit What You Don't Know

There is no way to know everything about type 1 diabetes. Understanding diabetes doesn't mean you have to know everything. It does help to be humble enough to admit when you don't know the answer and need help figuring it out. Faking it and guessing with diabetes rarely ends well and usually just makes you think you cannot handle it.

Step #4: Accept That You May Not Understand

We've all had those days where you can't get your blood sugar down no matter what you do. You count your carbs and take your insulin, and nothing happens. You open a new vial of insulin and change your pump site, but your blood sugar stays high. You're doing everything right, but diabetes refuses to cooperate. It makes absolutely no sense.

There are going to be times when you're not going to be able to figure out diabetes. You dive into your data, ask for help, and rack your brain for an explanation, but there isn't one. Accepting that your blood sugars are sometimes a mystery is part of understanding diabetes. If you understand that not understanding is part of the game with T1D, you'll have a much easier time handling the stress of T1D.

You Can't Handle What You Don't Manage

The second aspect of managing T1D that I want to focus on in this chapter is putting in the work. If you don't manage T1D, of course, it's going to be hard to handle. That's no surprise. I know it seems obvious, and it is. But I also know that your behavior probably doesn't always follow this simple logic.

Sometimes you may even throw this logic out the window. You convince yourself the only way you can handle the stress of T1D is to run from it. You get trapped in the *paradox of avoidance*.

The problem is, not managing T1D does nothing to help your stress. Running away from managing T1D makes it even harder to handle it. When you avoid doing what you know will help keep your blood sugar in range, you probably don't feel very well. And when you feel like you got hit by a bus because of high blood sugar, life with diabetes is rough.

But there's more.

When you don't manage your diabetes and then have a hard

time handling it, all you do is reinforce your belief that you can't cope with it. Life with T1D gets more challenging, and you blame yourself. You tell yourself that if you could deal with it, you would take care of yourself. You don't take care of yourself, and this is just more evidence that you can't handle it. Your avoidance becomes a self-fulfilling prophecy and ties you in a knot.

If you want to handle T1D, you must put in the work of managing it. Waiting until you think you can handle T1D to put in the work is a recipe for not being able to cope.

Doing the Work Makes T1D Easier to Handle

When you put in the work to manage T1D, it makes it easier to handle.

Slacking off on your diabetes management leads to higher blood sugars, so, of course, you're not going to feel great. On the flip side, doing the work will lead to more in-range blood sugars. You may not have perfect blood sugars (nobody with T1D does), but I promise you'll see an improvement. It would be almost impossible not to. When your blood sugars are lower, and you're able to get off the blood sugar roller coaster, you're going to feel better. You'll have more energy and focus.

Leaning into your diabetes management does much more than help you feel better. It also shows you what you're capable of. Sitting on the sidelines, you were reluctant to manage your diabetes because you were scared it would be too much work or your hard work wouldn't pay off. It was a mountain you thought was too steep to climb. Once you put in some work to manage your diabetes, you'll discover that yes, it's a lot of work, but you can find success. You'll also probably find that what you thought would be such a big deal is, with a bit of practice, something you can handle with ease.

At the core, managing diabetes is taking a set of rules and applying them to what's going on in your life at a particular time. The effort to manage diabetes gives you more freedom in your life, not less, because it means following a process. Unexpected challenges will come up, without a doubt. But when they do, you continue applying the rules to these new situations.

Will your blood sugars be perfect? Of course not. But they'll be more in range than if you didn't put in the work, and you'll think about them a lot less. Following the process and managing diabetes doesn't trap you in a world of stress. Instead, it frees you to live your life without having to think about diabetes any more than you need to. When you avoid managing your diabetes, you may think that you'll find the freedom you want and make diabetes easier to handle. But all avoidance does is make you think about diabetes even more. The choice is yours.

Strategies to Help You Engage with T1D

Now that you understand how by avoiding managing your diabetes you're making T1D harder to handle, not easier, hopefully, you're ready to dive in and engage with it. Of course, you'll want to work with your diabetes care team on the details, but here are some strategies to help you get started.

Strategy #1: Focus on Behaviors, Not Outcomes

It's easy to get frustrated and overwhelmed when your blood sugars are out of range, and you can't figure out the reason. It happens. T1D doesn't always play fair or make sense. Your CGM graph may not look pretty. However, that doesn't mean you aren't working hard to manage your blood sugars. We all know that you can do everything right, and your blood sugars still have a mind of their own.

Leaning into diabetes means focusing on your behaviors and not the outcomes, especially your blood sugar reading at any given time. Leaning in means engaging in the behaviors you know help you keep your blood sugars in range. Focusing on behaviors leads to outcomes. Focusing on results only leads to frustration and feeling overwhelmed.

If you're doing what you're supposed to do, you have my permission to call that a huge win!

Strategy #2: Take Steps, No Matter How Small

Diabetes management isn't one big task. It's a series of small, sometimes seemingly insignificant tasks that you're performing throughout the day. If you've been avoiding diabetes management for a long time, engaging doesn't have to mean doing a complete 180. Any step toward engaging with and managing your blood sugars, no matter how small, is a step in the right direction. The smallest actions can catapult you to some of the most significant victories. So just keep moving forward, even if it's by taking one small step at a time.

Strategy #3: Keep Moving Forward!

Do you ever feel like you take two steps forward and one step back with your diabetes management? You feel like you're doing so well for a couple of weeks, and then all of a sudden, you've slipped back into some of your old, unhealthy habits. Don't be too hard on yourself when this happens. Remember that progress with diabetes management rarely follows a straight path, and just because you've backtracked, it doesn't mean you haven't made progress. The trick here is as soon as you realize you've slipped back into your old habits, pick yourself up and keep moving forward.

Strategy #4: Progress, Not Perfection
I have some good news, and I have some bad news. I'll start with the bad news. No matter how much you work to manage diabetes, your blood sugars will never be perfect all the time. Now for the good news. No matter how much you work to manage diabetes, your blood sugars will never be perfect all the time.

I'm sure this news is not a surprise to you. I know it's a bit disappointing, but I also hope it takes some pressure off. Your goal is not to have perfect blood sugars. Achieving this goal simply isn't possible, and thinking you can sets you up for failure. Your goal is to keep making progress with diabetes, no matter how insignificant the progress feels. Forward momentum always results in positive change when it comes to managing T1D.

Managing T1D Helps You Handle T1D
Pushing diabetes under the rug doesn't help you handle it. Ignoring diabetes and pretending you don't need to take care of yourself only makes things worse. To get a grasp on T1D and deal with it effectively, you have to lean into your diabetes

management. Paying more attention to your diabetes, rather than less, will make it easier to handle. I promise.

CHAPTER 6 KEY TAKEAWAYS

- *The more you work to manage T1D, the easier T1D will be to handle.*

- *When you put in the work, your blood sugars will improve, and you will feel better.*

- *You will also see that the work you do matters.*

- *If you don't work to manage T1D, you'll get stuck in the belief that managing T1D is too tricky.*

- *In-range blood sugars are not the goal of managing T1D. Putting in the effort is the goal. In-range blood sugars will follow.*

Chapter 7

YOU CAN HANDLE UNCOMFORTABLE EMOTIONS

***You can handle** the challenging emotions T1D throws your way.*

I know this statement is bold, and you may not believe me right now. For a long time, you've probably been under the assumption that you can't handle the uncomfortable emotions that come with diabetes—frustration, exhaustion, worry, feeling overwhelmed, and even hopelessness.

I'll tell you right now that this assumption isn't correct, and I'm going to show you how you can handle these difficult emotions. You already can do it, and now all you need is a reminder, some skills, and a nudge forward to get you to the point where you can see it for yourself.

If you don't believe it's possible to handle your uncomfortable T1D emotions right now, that's okay. All I ask is that you're open to the possibility you may be wrong.

Remember to Be Honest with Yourself

Remember, to handle your challenging T1D emotions, you have to be honest with yourself. The feelings that come with T1D are challenging—there's no reason to pretend like they're not. Pretending diabetes doesn't bring up uncomfortable emotions is doing yourself a disservice. If you need to review all the challenging emotions that come along with diabetes, go back and reread Chapter 3.

You also have to be honest about your ability to control these emotions. No matter what you do, you will feel burned out, frustrated, and overwhelmed at times. You're human and T1D is stressful. When humans experience stress, uncomfortable feelings are never far behind. You have to accept that you will sometimes feel this way, and you can't always do much about it.

When you try to force these uncomfortable emotions to go away, it usually just intensifies your feelings and makes them even more uncomfortable. Trying to control your diabetes-driven emotions just makes them worse.

You may be asking where this leaves you. You know that diabetes comes with some challenging emotions, and there isn't much you can do to make them disappear. So what do you do?

You have to learn to live with these feelings and not let them get in your way. And trust me (and yourself) that you can handle them.

Handling the stress of living with T1D involves a set of skills that work together to help you come to a place of freedom with—not from— your challenging emotions. This chapter will teach you the three essential skills you need to deal with all the uncomfortable diabetes emotions (UDE) you've been working so hard to avoid.

Quick note ————————————————————————————

Remember, developing and maintaining skills around your emotional health with T1D takes work, and a lot of patience. Once you learn these skills, it takes ongoing practice to maintain them. This chapter will give you a roadmap to get you started. However, you can't expect just to check the box with your learning and be done. Developing the skills to handle your UDE takes more than learning about them on a theoretical basis. Mastering these skills takes active participation, engagement, and a willingness to stumble along the way. These are advanced skills, and you can expect to encounter challenges as you learn them.

Skill #1: Sit with the Discomfort

Yes, you read that correctly. I'm telling you that to handle your T1D-related emotions, you will need to not only accept them but also sit with them and not try to do anything to change them. You know that trying to avoid UDE only makes them worse, so the other option is to allow them to be there.

What does it mean to sit with discomfort on a practical level? And isn't this going to be, well, uncomfortable?

Let's break it down so you can see for yourself.

Be Mindful
The first step to sitting with discomfort is to be mindful. Mindfulness means paying attention to what's happening in the present moment without judgment. You're observing what's going on—what you're feeling, what you're thinking, what's happening around you. You're present. You simply notice what's going on for you without thinking about it or attaching any meaning to it.

Mindfulness takes continual practice. Our minds naturally wander away from the present moment and into the past or the future. We get lost in our thoughts. When this happens, our attention escapes from the here and now.

The present moment is where you feel overwhelmed, burned out, and frustrated with T1D. And, naturally, you want to escape these emotions. After all, they're uncomfortable, but escaping into the past or future doesn't work. It makes things worse.

Imagine you're in the park on a warm summer day enjoying a picnic lunch with your family. As you take a bite of your sandwich, the biggest bumblebee you have ever seen flies over and maneuvers around your area, doing touch-and-goes on your head. You hate bugs and have heard scary stories about bumblebees on sunny summer days, so your mind starts racing. You think about how awful it would be if you got stung. You think back to last summer when your friend got stung by a bee. All the while, your anxiety level shoots up as you get lost in your thoughts. And to top it off, you missed what your mom said she wants to do for her birthday later that month.

How do you practice mindfulness and stay connected to the present moment? Here are some tips to get started:

- **Find an anchor.** *Mindfulness is not about clearing your mind. It's about staying present with what's happening in your mind right now. You need an anchor to stay connected to the present moment. You can pay attention to your breath, use your hands or feet to ground you, or keep your gaze on an object. This anchor is something you can come back to when your mind wanders (and it will).*

- **Think of yourself as an observer of what's going on with you.** *In straightforward terms, describe it. For example, how do you feel emotionally—happy, sad, scared, timid? How do you feel physically— shaky, sweaty, heavy, energetic?*

- **Pay attention to your thoughts, without judging them.** *Your thoughts aren't good or bad. They just are. Label your thoughts as what they are— thoughts. Having a thought doesn't mean what you are thinking is true.*

How Mindfulness Works in Your Life with T1D
Think of all the times when something stressful happens with T1D. When these stressful things occur, my guess is your mind leaves the present moment, and you start

thinking. You can use mindfulness anytime something happens with T1D that makes you feel stressed.

Here are a few examples of when you can use mindfulness to deal with T1D stressors:

- *Your CGM goes off in the middle of a work meeting.*
- *You're at the gym, and you're self-conscious of your pump site visible on your abdomen.*
- *You pull out your insulin pen to bolus on a plane, and you're worried about what other people might think.*
- *Your significant other gets mad at you because your blood sugar is high after dinner.*
- *You're upset you had to cancel plans because you felt like you got hit by a bus after a bad low.*
- *You're feeling burned out after a day on a blood sugar roller coaster.*
- *Anytime you're feeling stressed out by diabetes!*

How Staying Present Helps You Handle T1D

When you're mindful, you notice what's happening, but you don't get wrapped up in it. You're still anxious, but you don't get lost in the anxiety. Instead, you stay present with it. When you're mindful, you also will have an easier time handling the stress of T1D.

This is because the present moment is the only place you can handle diabetes—you can't handle anything in your head. The only place you can manage challenging emotions is in the present moment. When you're unwilling to sit with the discomfort of diabetes, you're avoiding it. But that does nothing to make it go away, and it doesn't do anything to help you handle it. The only way to handle the tough stuff is to be present and lean into it. Also, the present moment is the easiest place to stay honest with yourself. This is where you can get to know your UDE on a real level instead of living in a world full of assumptions.

When you stay present, you show yourself that you can handle the stress. If you keep avoiding the stress, you'll never allow yourself to see what you're capable of. My guess is you'll surprise yourself.

Finally, staying in the present moment helps you see the difference between the things you can and cannot change about T1D. It's easier to handle the fact that there are some things about T1D you can't control if you can see there are things you can control.

REAL-LIFE T1D: JUSTIN

Justin told me about how he was feeling like a failure with T1D. Since he was diagnosed when he was 17, he's been searching for ways to make T1D easier to handle. With his diabetes educator's help, Justin has found ways to keep his blood sugars in a better range, but he still feels burned out, ashamed, and all alone no matter what he does. Whenever these feelings come up for Justin, he tends to isolate himself by playing video games so he doesn't have to face these feelings. He says the escape that video games provide is the only way he can cope. However, Justin also realizes that playing video games makes him feel even more alone and does nothing to relieve the pressure of diabetes. Everything he does to escape the present moment makes diabetes even more uncomfortable, making him want to escape even more.

Our work together focused on introducing Justin to a new way of thinking about T1D. He came to terms with the reality that diabetes may bring up some uncomfortable feelings for him at times. He started to notice these feelings and realized they were expected. He found that by sitting with these unpleasant feelings, their sting decreased pretty quickly. This was quite a change from the constant burden he had on his shoulders from always fighting them.

After learning mindfulness strategies and sitting with his difficult emotions, Justin found they became easier to handle. Paying attention to his experience in the present moment showed him what he was capable of and gave him the confidence he needed to lean into diabetes instead of running away from it.

— — —

Do you want to learn how to manage T1D mindfully?

Go to www.thediabetespsychologist.com/mindfulnessguide or scan the code on the next page to access guided exercises to help you integrate mindfulness into your life with T1D.

Remember, staying present with T1D is something you can always work toward. While you will never be able to be mindful in your life with T1D all the time (this is not possible for anyone), you can take steps to stay more present and make diabetes easier to handle in the process.

Skill #2: Let Go of Your Stories

Chapter 4 talked about how the stories you tell yourself about T1D are not always honest and how they tend to make your UDE more challenging than they need to be. These stories take something objectively stressful—like high blood sugar or feeling anxious about trying something new—and add unnecessary meaning, throwing fuel on the fire. The story made an already stressful situation worse because you added meaning that doesn't reflect reality.

I have some bad news and some good news about the stories you tell yourself about T1D.

First, I'll tell you the bad news.

You cannot stop these stories from brewing in your head. Humans are analytical creatures. We want to understand what's going on in our world, especially when parts of it are unexplainable. As you know, the experience of living with T1D doesn't always make a lot of sense. Often, our ability to understand the world and why things happen in our lives is useful. This skill helps us navigate challenges and keep ourselves safe.

But your ability to understand T1D is not perfect and has limitations. No matter how hard you try to figure it out, sometimes diabetes just makes no sense. However, people with T1D can be stubborn, and we don't give up that easily. The challenge is our efforts to try and make sense of the unexplainable can lead us astray. We create stories—most of which aren't true—about our diabetes in an effort to understand. These stories are going to appear whether you like it or not.

Now for the good news.

You have a choice about what to do with these stories. You may not be able to stop your stories from swirling around your head, but you can choose whether or not you pick them up and buy them. When you decide not to buy all your stories about diabetes, you set yourself up to handle the stress of T1D.

Do you like to shop at Target? I do (especially the day after Halloween for low snacks, but I digress)! Imagine if the next time you walk into your local Target, there is a sign on the door announcing a new store policy:

If you touch it, you have to buy it.

It sounds ridiculous, doesn't it? The whole reason you go to Target in the first place is that there are many things to look at. How will you be able to decide what you want to buy if you can't pick items up and look at them? I am a tactile person, and I like to touch things. Whenever I walk by a rack of clothes at Target, my hand is out brushing the fabric. If Target had this policy, I would be the proud owner of shirts of every size.

I'm sure you agree this policy is silly and defeats the whole purpose of shopping at Target. I'm also sure the powers that be at Target know this and would never consider making such a ridiculous rule. It would kill their business.

But, without knowing it, most of us have that same policy for our thoughts and stories. If a story about T1D shows up in your mind, you think must be true. And if it's true, you have to buy it. When these stories become part of how you think about diabetes, they make T1D hard to handle.

Quick note ————————————————————————

You will have stories about T1D that are accurate and that help you. Please, pick up these stories and buy them. Not all stories are negative or make the stress of T1D worse. Observing your stories helps you tell the difference between those that are helpful and those that aren't. That way, you can choose for yourself what stories you want to buy, rather than have the choice made for you.

REAL-LIFE T1D: CHELSEA

Chelsea loves being active, and she is also highly competitive. When her boyfriend suggested they train for a marathon last summer, she was all in. Over the past year, Chelsea has been working with a diabetes educator to dial in her diabetes management during exercise, and she was ready to take on this next challenge.

Chelsea found her groove, and everything was going well in her training. Then came the day for their 16-mile run. For breakfast, Chelsea ate some oatmeal and a banana and bolused for half the carbs. About ninety minutes later, she and her boyfriend set off on their run. Feeling good for the first three miles, she smiled, happy to be in the fresh air and feeling confident that her blood sugars would behave.

As they crossed mile 4, Chelsea glanced at her CGM and saw her blood sugar was trending down. No big deal, she thought and pulled out some gel to bring it back up. Then, about fifteen minutes later, she heard the alarm going off in her earphones.

Her blood sugar was 84 mg/dl, and she was crashing fast.

Chelsea motioned to her boyfriend that she needed to stop, and she sat down on the side of the road. Thirty minutes and four packets of gel later, with blood sugar still hovering around 80 mg/dl, Chelsea reluctantly told her boyfriend they needed to stop their run. She was physically exhausted from this unexpected low.

The stories started swirling around in Chelseas's head on the drive home from their aborted long run.

- *Diabetes is always holding me back.*

- *I'm never going to be able to be active like other*

people because of my stupid diabetes.

- *Diabetes put me at a competitive disadvantage.*

- *I'm so stupid for letting my blood sugar crash.*

- *I should have known better.*

By the time they got home, Chelsea was emotionally spent. She had bought all of these stories, and they took her to a dark place.

When I met with Chelsea several days later, I reminded her that she has no obligation to buy the stories she tells herself. And even when she does buy them, they have a generous return policy.

Letting Go of Your Stories Helps You Handle T1D

Not getting attached to your thoughts and stories is a great way to increase flexibility in your life with T1D. You may not be in control of these stories, but detaching from them can help ensure they don't control you.

Watching your stories is another way to practice mindfulness by letting them come and go without getting wrapped up in them. And if you do get tangled in one of the many stories you tell yourself about what living with T1D means for your life, the quickest way to disengage is to be aware of your entanglement and bring yourself back to the present moment. Watching your stories gives you the freedom and flexibility you need to handle the things about T1D that are stressful and make sure the additional meaning you put on them doesn't get in the way.

Here are some steps you can take to start letting go of your stories about diabetes.

Step #1: Recognition
Good news! By reading this book, you already have started to recognize that you tell yourself stories about T1D, which increases your stress and makes it harder to handle T1D. You also may have begun to identify the types of stories you tend to tell yourself.

Pro tip: *Even though every story may be slightly different, they likely will have similar themes.*

The first step to watching your diabetes stories is recognizing these stories exist and that they can increase your stress. Since you probably have been telling yourself some version of these stories for a while now, they have become part of how you think about yourself and your diabetes. After some time, you assume your stories are accurate and take them at face value. Calling out your stories for what they are (they're just stories!) helps you start to observe, rather than buy, them.

Exercise
Take a minute and list the types of stories you tend to tell yourself about T1D. Identifying the common themes of the stories you've told yourself in the past will help you notice your stories in the future.

Complete these sentences to help you get started:

- *Diabetes makes me...*

- *Having T1D means I am...*

- *When my blood sugar is out of range, it means I...*

- *It's _____ that I have T1D.*

Step #2: Observation

In this step, you pay attention to your stories about T1D as they come to life in your head. This is where you get to practice your mindfulness skills.

Be sure to go back and read about the anatomy of a story in Chapter 4.

Pro tip: *You may have a hard time identifying your stories in the moment. This is common and doesn't mean you're doing anything wrong. If you're having trouble observing your stories, try working backward. Start with your emotions. When you experience a negative feeling with T1D, there's usually a story behind the emotion. Identify what you're feeling, and then ask yourself what's making you feel that way. There is typically a story hiding in there somewhere waiting to be uncovered.*

Exercise

When something challenging happens in your life with T1D, whether you have a run-of-the-mill low blood sugar or you end up in the hospital with DKA, stories form. As you start to observe your stories about T1D, ask yourself the following questions:

- *Are there specific things that trigger my stories?*

- *How do I go about meaning-making with my stories?*

- *Do my stories take me to the past or the future?*

- *How do these stories impact my diabetes management and my quality of life?*

Step #3: Detachment

Watching your stories means recognizing and accepting that there are some things about diabetes that you can't control. And it means you have to let go of trying to understand what cannot be understood. It means letting go of the unhelpful stories you've been holding onto. This is one of the most challenging parts of the process.

Detachment doesn't mean trying to push the story out of your mind. That's not possible. Detachment means not buying the story. It means not grabbing onto it simply because it appeared. It means noticing the stories you tell yourself but not engaging with them. And when you do start to engage with them, it means putting your hands up and letting go as soon as you realize what you're doing.

When you detach from your stories, you take off your gloves and stop wrestling with them. This process can feel messy because it means letting go of the illusion that you can control your stories around T1D. However, when you let go of your firm grip, you let go of control. You also take power away from your story, which gives you more freedom and flexibility. If anything can help you handle the stress of T1D, it's freedom and flexibility.

Once you realize you're telling yourself a story about T1D, name it. Labeling a story for what it is can take power away from it and help you detach. Here are a couple of simple things you can do to identify the stories you tell yourself about T1D.

Call Out Your Story
Whenever a story appears in your thoughts, say to yourself, "That's just a story, and I don't have to buy it." This simple reminder is a great way to start letting go of your stories.

Use These Words
When you're speaking to other people (or yourself) about T1D, and you catch yourself talking like you've already bought this story, put these words in front of what you're saying: "I'm telling myself a story that (insert story here)." For example, if you start telling someone, or yourself, that you're never going to get your blood sugars under control, you can say: "I'm telling myself a story that I'm never going to get my blood sugars under control." Do you see how adding that simple (and accurate) preface takes the wind out of the story's sail?

Talk to Your Story
I know this sounds silly, and it is. But sometimes, you just need to lighten the mood to detach from your story. When you notice one of your familiar stories about T1D making an appearance in your life, say hello! Let the story know that you see it, and be sure to make it clear that you don't have

time to talk right now because you have more important things you need to do. Here is a script you can use:

> *"Hey there, story about (insert a brief description of the story here)! I want to let you know that I see you stopped by today for a visit. You're welcome to stick around, but, unfortunately, I don't have time to pay attention to you right now. I'm moving forward in my life, so you're going to be on your own! Enjoy your day!"*

Let Go of Your Story

Grab a tissue and look at it. Imagine that this piece of paper is your story about what T1D means about you. Hold out your hand with your palm up and let your story land. Now grab your story and hold on tight. Look what happened. Your story is now a part of you, and it will be hard to pry out. Now grab another tissue and do the same thing. Let it land on your open hand. But instead of grabbing onto it and holding it tight, just let it be. The story is still there, but all you're doing is noticing it's there. You're not engaging with it and not holding onto it. Your interaction with the story completely changed your relationship with it. You were able to detach from it. Next time one of your stories appears, treat it like this tissue. Let it land, but do not engage with it.

Step #4: Practice and Patience

Learning to recognize, identify, and detach from your stories about T1D is not something that is just going to happen. It takes practice and patience. You've probably been telling yourself these stories for a while now, so buying them feels natural. It's just what you do. The only way to detach from these stories is to get out of your comfort zone and practice interacting with them differently. When you recognize your mind has wandered into an unhelpful story about what T1D means about you, practice noticing it without engaging with it.

As you practice detaching from your stories about T1D, try to be patient with yourself. Old habits die hard. Be kind to yourself if you find yourself engaging with and buying your stories about diabetes (and it will happen). As soon as you notice this happening, take steps to detach from the story and try not to beat yourself up. Remember, the urge to beat yourself up will come from telling yourself a story.

Skill #3: See Yourself as More than T1D

Imagine you're sitting on a beautiful beach. The water is crystal clear, the sun is shimmering on the water, and everybody is having a great time—except you. You're holding a giant beach ball in front of your face. You can't see any of the beauty around you because the beach ball is blocking your view. All you can see is the beach ball.

The next day, your mom asks about your day at the beach, and you tell her you didn't have any fun. You tell her the beach is boring, and there isn't much to see. You didn't see any water at the beach, and you didn't see the sun. When she asks you to describe what you could see, you tell her the only thing to see for miles was a beach ball.

I know this story sounds ridiculous, however, we often see diabetes in the same way we see the beach ball. It is all-consuming. It takes up our headspace. You can't see what's going on around you because diabetes is blocking the view.

If T1D is indeed all-consuming, there's no doubt it's going to be hard to handle. If something is all-consuming, it's always in your line of sight, and you can't see or think about anything else. It steals your ability to enjoy things in life.

And, of course, diabetes is always going to be there. Unlike a beach ball, you can't leave it at home or put it in the trash.

But back to the beach ball. What if, instead of holding it so close to your face, you stretched out your arms? The beach ball is still in your line of sight, and it's blocking part of your view, but now you can see a lot more of the beach.

Try doing the same thing with the stress around T1D. See your life in the context of your diabetes and not entirely consumed by diabetes. It's there, and there may be times when it does get in your way. But it's not the only thing in your line of sight.

I know it may not feel like it, but there's much more to you than type 1 diabetes. When you can recognize that T1D helps explain, but doesn't define you, it will be much easier to handle the stress of diabetes.

I know there are some days when you feel like the burden of diabetes will never end. You feel like the frustration and overwhelming emotions you have because of diabetes are tattooed on your arm. These challenges are a permanent part of you, and there is no chance they'll ever change.

When you're in the forest of those emotions, it's hard to see a way out. It's like you've always been there, and you'll always be there.

When you feel this way, take an honest look and ask yourself how accurate this feeling is. The reality is your experience with T1D is dynamic. It is constantly changing, even when you don't notice the change.

Yes, you have T1D. Your pancreas no longer produces insulin, and until we have a cure (and I'm not holding my breath), this is not going to change. But that isn't what I'm talking about here. What's constantly changing is your experience of living with diabetes. This includes how you feel physically and emotionally. It includes your blood sugar readings and trends. It even includes how motivated you are to take care of yourself.

These experiences are never the same for long. At times you may be doing really well; at other times you may be struggling; and at still other times you may be somewhere in between. If your experience with T1D is constantly changing, then there's no way for what you're experiencing now to define you. Whatever is happening for you now explains your current experience and nothing more.

But more importantly, whatever you're experiencing at a specific moment in your life with T1D doesn't change you. It doesn't leave a permanent mark on you and doesn't change who you are. When you believe what you're experiencing changes the core of who you are, it makes T1D harder to handle.

There's a part of you that is stable. This part has always been with you and isn't going away anytime soon. This is the core of who you are, and no matter what happens in your life, that part of you isn't going to change. You may not always notice because your current feelings overshadow it, but that core is always there.

What about who you are is stable and not going to change anytime soon? Here are some examples to get you thinking:

- *The color of your eyes*

- *Your (natural) hair color*

- *Your role in your family (for example, you are a mother, father, daughter, son)*

- *Aspects of your personality (kind, adventurous, curious, etc.)*

- *Your pancreas doesn't work as it should (you have diabetes)*

- *Where you're from*

- *Your values*

There also are aspects of your life that are constantly changing. But when they change, these things don't alter the core of who you are. They only change what you're experiencing right now. Sometimes you choose to make these changes, and sometimes they just happen. Some of them may be changes you want; some you don't.

What about your experience is continually changing? Here are some examples to get you thinking:

- *What you are wearing*
- *Your blood sugar*
- *How burned out you feel*
- *Your anxiety*
- *Your energy level*
- *Your mood*
- *Your motivation*
- *Your schedule*
- *All your thoughts about T1D*

Your current experience impacts your quality of life, however it is constantly changing. It will get better in the future, and it probably also will get worse. The one thing you do know is that it will never be the same for very long.

Your current experience flavors you, but it does not define you.

What does any of this have to do with your ability to handle the stress of T1D?

Do you have a mixing bowl in your kitchen? One of those sturdy bowls you've had forever and use almost every day?

This mixing bowl is you. It's the part of you that's stable. This mixing bowl was made to last and to stand up to whatever gets thrown inside of it.

You put all kinds of ingredients into this mixing bowl, and these "ingredients" are what's happening for you right now.

No matter what you put in the mixing bowl, the bowl stays the same. Sometimes there may be delicious food in the bowl. There also may be times when what's in the bowl is disgusting. The contents of the bowl are constantly changing. The ingredients all get mixed, new ones are added, others are taken out, and the bowl takes a beating. But whatever you do, it doesn't change the core of the bowl. The contents may be a mess, but the bowl remains the same. There is nothing you can do to change the bowl.

A part of you is the same person you were before you were diagnosed with T1D. I know it may not always feel like it, but there is so much more to you than your diabetes. Once you can see that diabetes hasn't changed the core of who you are and that there is more to you than diabetes, it becomes easier to handle. T1D still is going to suck at times, but just because diabetes sucks, it doesn't have to define who you are. You see that there is more to you than your T1D, and this perspective makes diabetes easier to handle.

REAL-LIFE T1D: JAKE

Since he was diagnosed with T1D six years ago, Jake has felt burdened by his diabetes. He describes T1D as having a weight superglued to his body. Jake talks about how diabetes invades every aspect of his life and how it has permanently changed him. He misses the old Jake, convinced the adventurous, carefree guy he was before T1D appeared in his life is gone forever.

Jake just returned from a three-week trip to Europe. He came to see me, and his bitterness started pouring out. Jake told me about how diabetes had ruined his trip. Several days, he woke up with sky-high blood sugar and had to sit out that day's excursions because he wasn't feeling well. He went low most days in the late afternoon, so he had to stop, and everyone had to wait for him while his blood sugar came up.

When he returned, all Jake could talk about was how challenging the trip was for him because he was on a blood sugar roller coaster all week. Diabetes was at the front of his mind, and he couldn't see past it. The weight was still superglued to his shoulder, and he was convinced that there would never be a time when the stress of diabetes was not going to be in his way.

What can you do to start seeing yourself as more than your diabetes? Here are some steps you can take to get started.

Step #1: Make a List

Some things aren't evident to us unless they're right in front of our faces. As you know from the beach ball we talked about earlier in this chapter, it's easy to let T1D be front and center and block your view of all the other parts of your life. To bring them back into view, you have to know they are there and look for them. Making a list is the first step.

Take a pen and paper and write down the things about yourself that aren't changing. These are what have been with you for as long as you can remember and won't change in the foreseeable future. Think personality, interests, family.

Next, write down some things you're experiencing right now but that aren't permanent. A word of caution as you look for your experiences. When you're in the middle of them, sometimes your experiences—especially the challenging ones—feel like they're part of you. One trick is to put the words "right now" and "next year" at the end of the phrase and see what it sounds like. For example:

I have T1D right now. I will have T1D next year. You can be confident that both statements are accurate.

I am feeling burned out by T1D right now. I will feel burned out by T1D next year. You know the first statement is accurate because that's what you're experiencing right now. The second statement may be true, but it's also possible you won't feel burned out next year. You won't know for sure until then. And even if you do feel burned out next year, it's likely it won't look the same as it does right now.

Step #2: Write Down What's Going on Beyond T1D

Now write down all the things going on in your life that have nothing to do with T1D. For example, maybe you're going on a trip next month that you're excited about. Or maybe your daughter is starting kindergarten next year. Are you reading any good books? Is there a new television show you're bingeing? Are you in a new relationship you're excited about?

It doesn't matter what's going on in your life, even if it's not exciting. Write down whatever you can think of, as long as it does not directly involve diabetes.

Step #3: Practice, Practice, Practice!

Remember what you wrote in step #2 the next time you're overwhelmed and feel like diabetes consumes your thoughts.

First, you want to remind yourself that what you're feeling right now is not permanent. It's not part of who you are. It's only part of what you're experiencing right now, and you know it won't last forever. It can and will change.

When you feel overwhelmed, acknowledge your feelings and recognize what else is happening around you. Move your overwhelming emotions away from your face so you can see and experience other things along with whatever is going on for you right now.

Allowing things other than your current experience with T1D into your line of sight takes practice. It's probably not part of your routine, but with some practice, you'll be able to see the challenges you're having with T1D for what they really are. These struggles are part of your everyday experience and not what defines you.

With this new perspective, you'll start to see that even though T1D sucks sometimes, you have the ability to handle it.

CHAPTER 7 KEY TAKEAWAYS

- *You can handle the uncomfortable emotions that come with living with T1D.*

- *Handling your uncomfortable diabetes emotions (UDE) involves a set of skills that you can develop. These skills include:*

  - *Learning to sit with discomfort.*

  - *Letting go of your stories.*

  - *Seeing yourself as more than a person with T1D.*

- *When you can handle the uncomfortable emotions T1D throws your way, they'll still be there, but they won't get in your way or bother you as much.*

Chapter 8

LEAD WITH ACTION

CONFIDENCE IS THE EXPERIENCE OF
SUCCESS REPEATED TIME AFTER TIME.

—DENIS MORTON

EVERYTHING WE'VE TALKED about so far has led us to this chapter. The way you will know you can handle the stress of T1D is when you lead with action.

Remember the real reason you're having a difficult time handling diabetes. It's not the stories you tell yourself about what diabetes means about you. It's not the uncomfortable emotions or the stress of T1D.

You're having a hard time handling diabetes because of how it gets in your way. The stress of T1D stops you from doing the things in your life that you want to do. You feel like you can't be spontaneous. You have a hard time traveling or doing outdoor activities. You think T1D makes you less attractive to a potential partner, so you may not even put yourself out there and try to meet someone new. You feel like diabetes boxes you in and prevents you from the possibility of stepping out of your comfort zone.

Diabetes makes you feel stuck, and you do not want to be stuck. Feeling stuck sucks, and feeling stuck makes T1D more challenging to handle.

I would be willing to bet that it would be much easier for you if T1D wasn't in your way and did not stop you from doing what you want in your life.

This is exactly what it means to handle T1D.

Handling something means nothing more than being capable of carrying a heavy load. It doesn't mean it will be easy to carry or that it will be fun to deal with. But just because something is not easy or fun doesn't mean it has to stop you. Once you get some experience and see you can do it, things almost always become more manageable.

What It Means to Lead with Action

Have you ever said to yourself, I will do ABC when I feel XYZ?

We say these types of things all the time. For example...

- *I'll start paying attention to my blood sugars when I'm feeling more motivated.*

- *I'll take the entire bolus for the carbs I'm eating when I feel confident that I won't go low.*

- *I'll take my son skiing when I'm not feeling so overwhelmed with T1D.*

Pay attention to the message you're sending yourself when you say these things. You're telling yourself that your feelings are in charge of your behavior. You have given your emotions about T1D control over what you can do in your life.

When you think this way, you are leading with your emotions. Hopefully, the day will come when you feel motivated, confident, and not so overwhelmed, and then you'll be able to take action. But you don't know when, or if, that will ever happen. Leading with your emotions leaves you feeling stuck. No matter how much you try, you can't just snap your fingers and change how T1D makes you feel. Emotions, especially the tough ones, just don't work that way.

When you lead with action, you turn the tables and take power away from your emotions. Leading with action means deciding what you want to do and then doing it, no matter how you feel. You lead with your behavior, and your emotions follow along, not the other way around.

REAL-LIFE T1D: TOM

Tom came to see me because he was having intense anxiety anytime he thought his blood sugar might be dropping. His anxiety had gotten so bad that he was having a hard time leaving his house. Tom worked in construction and getting to work every day was a struggle.

Tom was passionate about surfing, and his friends were planning the surfing trip of a lifetime. They had rented a boat off the coast of Indonesia, and they were going to live on and surf off the boat for ten days. Tom had paid for the trip and was looking forward to it, but his anxiety was getting in the way, and he was seriously considering telling his friends he couldn't go.

I saw Tom a couple of times, and then he disappeared. About a month later, he called and asked if he could come to see me again. My instinct told me he was going to confess he bailed on the trip at the last minute.

My instinct was wrong.

Instead, Tom sat in my office and told me all about his trip and what a great time he had. I stopped him and asked what had happened to his anxiety. His response was something I will never forget.

He said…

"I walked on the plane, and I had my surfboard under one arm and my anxiety under the other arm. I carried them both with me."

What Tom did is precisely what I mean when I talk about leading with action.

Before working with me, Tom was letting his anxiety dictate whether he could go on the surfing trip. When his panic was there, he thought he would have to cancel. When his anxiety eased, Tom was hopeful he could go. He was at the mercy of his anxiety.

Then something shifted for him. He realized that he could do what he wanted to do, even with his anxiety.

Would it be annoying? *Of course.*

Did it have to be debilitating? *No.*

Could he handle it? *He discovered that yes, he could!*

I love this story because it showed Tom what was possible, even while experiencing something that sucks, like anxiety about low blood sugar.

The same thing is true for you in your life with T1D. You can lead with action and carry the parts of T1D that suck with you. There is nothing else you can do with them.

What T1D-related emotions can you carry with you and still do what you want in life? Here are some examples...

- *Anxiety*
- *Burnout*
- *Frustration*
- *Anger*
- *Fear*
- *Lack of motivation*
- *So many more!*

Leading with action sounds simple. All you have to do is smile and face your T1D-related fears, right? Then you'll discover that all those things you were scared of really aren't all that scary after all. Life and T1D will be easy!

Again, I have some bad news and some good news.

The bad news is, leading with action isn't that simple. If it were easy, you would have started doing it long ago, and you probably never would have picked up this book. Leading with action is not straightforward because T1D is hard, and you have a lot of things getting in your way, including:

- *Spiraling thoughts about your ability to lead with action.*

- *Feelings of being overwhelmed from the stress of T1D and hopelessness that you'll ever be able to ease the burden.*

- *Concern about how others see you.*

Type 1 diabetes puts some real barriers to changing your behaviors in your way, and these barriers are real. It is probably not your first instinct to lead with action, and the thought of trying to overcome these barriers is a big reason.

Here's the good news. You can lead with action! Right now, you have all the tools you need to lead with action and let your emotions follow along. Up to this point, everything in this book has been about giving you the tools you need to take this step and not let fear get in the way of action.

T1D sucks. If you are honest with yourself, taking action and doing what you want to do in your life will probably be uncomfortable.

But you can handle it.

Not long after I was diagnosed with T1D, I jumped out of a perfectly good airplane. I not only survived to tell you about it, but looking back, it was one of my most memorable adventures. Although most of that day is a blur, there are several things about the experience that I vividly recall more than 20 years later.

The first thing I remember is my trepidation leading up to it. The thought of jumping out of a plane was exciting in theory and terrifying in reality. My heart and mind raced, and my hands shook visibly as the plane lifted off the ground.

I remember how I felt immediately after I jumped (actually, the instructor strapped to my back pushed me out). It was exhilarating, and all the fear I felt before the jump was gone.

My anxiety wrapped up in anticipation of taking action didn't match the reality of my experience once I took action. The fear I felt could have easily gotten in my way and prevented me from skydiving (and to be quite honest, it likely would have if I had not been with a group of close friends who never would've let me hear the end of it). But I'm glad it didn't. The anticipation of how scary it was going to be was so much worse than the reality of it. If I'm honest, my expectation and the reality were nowhere close to being the same.

The same thing happens in your behavior with T1D.

People tell me all the time how much they dread changing their pump site or CGM sensor. They put off checking their blood sugar or bolusing because it feels like a monumental task. The thought of taking a large dose of insulin feels overwhelming. They may not even consider exercising because the fear of going low stops them in their tracks.

When you finally take action either out of necessity or desire, you almost always will realize that what you were putting off was not nearly as burdensome, time-consuming, or scary as you thought it would be. You found the anticipation of taking action was much worse than the action itself.

Your thoughts were getting in your way. These thoughts lead to fear, anxiety, and even dread. Once you navigate around your thoughts and take action, you find the thing you put off was not that hard—and certainly not as hard as you had made it out to be.

But the only way for you to know how hard it is to do it is to lead with action.

You aren't going to feel confident until you allow yourself to succeed. And until you find success, taking action is going to be uncomfortable and even scary. However, unless you are willing to be uncomfortable, you will never find confidence with T1D. Leading with action is the only way for you to find the confidence you're looking for.

Four Steps to Lead with Action

How do you get started leading with action? Here is a step-by-step process to lead with action in your life with T1D.

Step #1: Be Intentional

You will not be able to lead with action without intention. You won't just wake up one day and start doing things you've been avoiding. As much as you wish this would be the case, it just isn't. You have to decide what you want to do and commit to doing it, no matter how you feel.

With T1D, commitment trumps anxiety. Once you commit to taking action, you're more than halfway there because you have moved from talking to planning. Talk is easy—putting a plan in place makes it real. Your commitment takes your desire and moves it forward in a very real way.

Exercise

Be intentional and commit to leading with action in your life with T1D. To get started, take out a piece of paper and write your answers to the following questions:

- *What exactly do you want to do?*

- *When do you want to do it?*

- *What might get in your way of taking action?*

- *What will you do to deal with that barrier?*

- *How will you know you've been successful?*

- *How are you going to hold yourself accountable?*

Step #2: Take Action

This step is where the rubber hits the road. You're going to put your plan into action and follow through on your commitment to yourself.

Yes, you're going to be scared. *Don't let your fear drive your behavior.*

Yes, you're going to want to back out. *Don't let this desire drive your behavior.*

Yes, you're going to have second thoughts. *Don't let your thoughts drive your behavior.*

Diabetes sucks, and you can handle it. And the way you're going to handle it right now is by not letting it get in your way. Remember, if the stress of T1D doesn't stop you from doing what you want to do, it won't be that big of a deal.

You have all the tools you need to lead with action. Now is the time to get out of your heart and let your head decide what you're going to do. You may be doing it scared, but you have to do it.

REAL-LIFE T1D: SARA

Sara has always been self-conscious about her body. Even before being diagnosed with T1D at the beginning of her senior year of high school, she did not like how she looked. And in Sara's mind, diabetes has taken her lack of confidence about her body to the next level.

She always seems worried about something with her body. In some seasons, it's her weight. In others, it's the scar tissue from hundreds of pump sites she has used over the past seven years. Right now, the focus of her angst is on the devices themselves. She wears a pump and a CGM, and they make her feel like a cyborg.

Most of the time, Sara figures out how to keep people from seeing the diabetes tech stuck to her body. But she's going on vacation to the beach for a week with some girlfriends and their significant others, and if she wants to wear a bathing suit—and in theory, she does—her pump and CGM will have nowhere to hide.

Sara was so worried about having people she just met see her diabetes devices that she worked out a plan to avoid going to the beach, or if she had to go to the beach, how she could stay covered. At one point, she even thought about backing out of the trip altogether.

As we talked about her worries, I reminded Sara that she could lead with action. She was probably never going to feel confident enough to wear a swimsuit and show off her pump and CGM. However, feeling self-conscious and lacking confidence did not have to stop her. For Sara, leading with action meant separating her self-deprecating thoughts and feelings from her behavior. She knew she would be uncomfortable, but she decided it was important to do it anyway.

So Sara led with action. She went to the beach, and she wore her devices. She decided to hold her head high and act as normal as possible. It turns out, what happened was not exactly what Sara was expecting. She was very nervous, and she felt more self-conscious than she ever had before. But to her surprise, no one noticed her devices, or if they did, they didn't say anything to her about them. She also realized that even though she was self-conscious the first day, she noticed it less and less as the week went on. By the last day, she put on her swimsuit without even thinking about people seeing her devices.

When she got home, she noticed other things about her body that she didn't like very much. She was still self-conscious, but after her week at the beach, she had some good evidence that she could lead with action, and her thoughts about diabetes and her body didn't have to stop her from doing anything. And in Sara's book, that's a huge win.

Step #3: Debrief Yourself
After you step forward and lead with action, always do a quick debriefing to look back at what you learned from the experience. Here are some questions to ask yourself:

- *How do you feel after you lead with action?*
- *Did your fears come true? Was the experience as uncomfortable as you thought it would be?*
- *What about leading with action was difficult?*
- *How has the emotional burden of T1D changed?*
- *Will it be easier for you to lead with action next time?*

You want to learn from the experience of leading with action, so you start to notice your successes, identify areas for improvement, and gain more confidence that you can handle the stress of T1D.

Step #4: Rinse and Repeat
Leading with action is not a one-time event. You'll continue

to lead with action for the rest of your life. You'll keep pushing yourself forward and out of your comfort zone.

When you lead with action, some things will get easier. But new things will pop up, and your thoughts and your emotions will get in the way of these actions. It may feel like you're playing a game of whack-a-mole with your feelings. However, once you nail the skill of leading with action and taking your emotions along with you, anything is possible with T1D. You just need to keep your commitment to lead with action, confident that you have the tools you need to do it.

— — —

Do you want help making a commitment to lead with action in your life with T1D?

Go to www.thediabetespsychologist.com/leadwithaction or scan the code below to download a free tool that will guide you through the process.

— — —

———— CHAPTER 8 KEY TAKEAWAYS ————

- *The only way to show yourself you can handle the stress of T1D is by leading with action.*

- *Leading with action with T1D means deciding what you want to do and doing it, no matter what emotions get in your way.*

- *There are four steps to leading with action in your life with T1D:*

    - *Be intentional*

    - *Take action*

    - *Debrief yourself*

    - *Rinse and repeat*

- *Don't forget, leading with action is an ongoing process in your life with T1D.*

Chapter 9

DON'T DO IT ALONE

*ASKING FOR HELP ISN'T WEAK,
IT IS A GREAT EXAMPLE OF HOW
TO TAKE CARE OF YOURSELF.*

—CHARLIE BROWN

I TELL MY patients, without exception, that I want them to find ways to get support from other people as part of their treatment with me. This includes friends and family, as well as other people with T1D.

And I'm going to tell you the same thing.

No one should have to do T1D on their own.

Getting the support you need from both other people with T1D and people close to you in your life will help you handle the stress of living with diabetes. Everyone with T1D needs and deserves support. It should be no surprise that lack of support makes T1D harder to handle.

If you feel alone with T1D, this doesn't mean you can't handle it. A critical part of handling T1D is embracing that you should never do T1D by yourself and knowing when to ask for support. Seeking support doesn't mean you can't handle T1D. Quite the opposite. It is a sign of strength.

Types of Support

Social support for people with T1D includes so much more than having someone who will listen to you vent about your blood sugar roller coasters. There are many faces of support, and they are all essential aspects of handling the stress of T1D. Here are some of the most important types of support that people with diabetes need:

Emotional

With all the pressure that comes with T1D, you're going to need people who can be a shoulder to cry on, who can cheer you up, and people who you can vent to when it feels like no matter what you do, your blood sugars are not going your way.

Logistical

This support includes getting rides to doctor appointments, figuring out the best way to order diabetes supplies, and navigating the maze of insurance coverage. Living with T1D can be a logistical nightmare, and we can all use support in figuring it out.

Physical

There are times when you just don't feel well, and you need help doing things. For example, when your blood sugar is low, you may need someone to help you get glucose. Or, if your blood sugar is high and you need to rest, you may need someone to help you with chores around the house, like taking care of your kids.

Financial

Diabetes is expensive. The price of insulin alone is a lot, and when you add on diabetes technology and expenses like co-pays for doctor appointments, the financial burden of T1D can be overwhelming. If you can't afford even the essential tools you need to manage T1D, you'll have difficulty handling it. Many folks need financial support from family, friends, or the health care system to help them manage diabetes, stay healthy, and still make ends meet.

Who You Need Support From

You need support from a variety of people, including:

Friends and Family

You are around your friends and family the most, so they are the most obvious folks to support you. Whether you need someone to listen to you vent about your blood sugars, someone to help you figure out how many carbs are in your dinner, or anything else, these are probably the first people you'll go to when you need support. Hopefully, they also are the most willing and able to give you the support you need.

Your Health Care Team

Your diabetes care team is there to help ensure you have what you need to keep your blood sugars in range. But, hopefully, you have a team that can support you in dealing with the stress of diabetes. These are the folks who understand the mechanics of diabetes, so they can help you figure out patterns in your blood sugars and make suggestions to help avoid big spikes. A good diabetes team also understands the emotional landmines of T1D and can support you in navigating around these challenges.

Others with T1D

These are the folks who know first-hand what it's like to live with diabetes every day. They understand exactly what it feels like to have high and low blood sugars. They know what it is like when people say ignorant things about diabetes. These people are your tribe, the people who speak the language of T1D. Others with T1D are certainly not your only avenue for support, but they are a necessary component of your support system. You need to know they are there and that you can call on them if you need something that only someone else with T1D can provide—an extra vial of insulin, a knowing glance when your CGM alarm goes off, someone who knows you're not on drugs when you talk about being high. Someone who gets exactly how you feel.

How to Get the Support You Need

The simple answer is you need to ask for the support you need. If you don't ask for help, people won't know what you need.

As people with T1D, we need support from the people in our lives. But getting the help you need isn't always easy. My bet is the people in your life want to be supportive, but they may not know how.

When T1D gets stressful and you have a hard time with it, you think everyone around you knows exactly how you feel. Let me tell you a secret. They probably don't have a clue.

And even if they do know how you feel, they probably have no idea what they can do to help you.

Before you can ask for the support you need, you need to know exactly what support will be most helpful for you. If this question stumps you, you're not alone. Identifying what you need from others to support you with your diabetes and make T1D easier to handle can feel overwhelming.

You probably know you need something, but you have no idea what that something looks like. If this sounds like you, go back to the beginning of this book and look at all the reasons why T1D sucks for you. Hopefully, after reading this book, you're having an easier time handling the challenging parts of T1D, but there are probably some areas where you're still struggling. As you work to define the support you need, focus on your biggest pain points.

Write down these pain points so they are clear in your mind. Be sure to include what each pain point is, why it's such a big challenge for you right now, and how you'll know when it has gotten easier for you.

Pro tip: *If you're struggling but are still having difficulty identifying your pain point, this confusion is your pain point! You can ask the people in your life to support you in figuring out why you're struggling so much with T1D, and then you can work together to find ways they can help you.*

Once you're clear on the areas of your life with T1D where you can use support, the next step is to identify the specific people, or type of person, who can support you. I encourage you to think outside the box here and not limit yourself to people you already know—more on that in a minute.

Next, start matching the support you need with the people, or type of people, who can offer you this support. Don't worry if you can't find a perfect match for all the support you need. Once you open the door and invite people to help you, the gaps in support will fill in on their own.

Now comes the most challenging part—asking for the specific support you need. You're probably feeling nervous about putting yourself out there and making your needs known. This feeling is normal. But remember, you live with T1D, and you have good evidence that you can handle uncomfortable situations, so I have no doubt that you can do this.

When asking for support from others, be clear and direct. I know you think everyone should know exactly what you need, but the people in your life aren't mind readers, and they may not even know you need help. Or if they do know you need assistance, they probably have no clue what help you need. They may think they know, but most likely, they're wrong.

You need to tell them precisely what you need and how they can help you. If you don't, they won't know, and you won't get the right kind of support. Being direct and guiding people in how they can support you can feel uncomfortable, but a little discomfort for a lot of support is nothing you can't handle.

Here are some statements to get you started asking for support with diabetes:

- *It would really help me if you got me some juice when my blood sugar is low.*

- *Please ask me how I am doing with diabetes burn-out every once in a while.*

- *I would appreciate it if you would stop asking me about my blood sugar every time I see you.*

- *One thing that would help is to remind me to pre-bolus when we are 20 minutes out from eating.*

- *My roller coaster blood sugars are making me feel overwhelmed. I could use your help figuring out what is going on and how I can stay grounded.*

- *Please don't treat me like I'm broken. Yes, I have T1D, but I can do everything you can do. It's not helpful when you say things like that, and I don't feel supported.*

A note about boundaries

You probably noticed the statements above include requests for what you want and don't want people to do to support you. Both types of requests are equally valid.

A boundary is a way to help you define what you're comfortable with and how you would like to be treated by others. Boundaries let you accept support that helps you and don't allow gestures that people think are helpful into your life. We all know the type of support that people think is valuable is not beneficial at all times.

Setting good, appropriate boundaries is crucial to be clear with others about how they can support you. Sometimes, this support means backing off rather than leaning in.

I am sure there have been times in your life when friends have tried to support you with T1D, but in reality, all they're doing is crossing a boundary. Good boundaries are essential for healthy relationships. For people with T1D, boundaries are even more crucial.

Do you notice people crossing boundaries around T1D with you? Here are some examples of what it looks like when people cross T1D-related boundaries:

- *Your teacher questions you about what you should or shouldn't be eating.*

- *Your best friend demands to know your blood sugar.*

- *Your coach tells you that you're not working hard enough with T1D*

- *Your wife ignores you when you tell her you need her support when you feel overwhelmed with your high blood sugars.*

- *Your endocrinologist makes a snide comment about how much insulin you take.*

- *Your dietician tells you what you can and cannot eat.*

- *Your diabetes educator threatens you with future complications if you don't listen to what he says.*

- *No one on your diabetes care team bothers to ask how you're doing and what support you need.*

As you tell people how they can best support you in dealing with the emotional challenges of T1D, remember the vital role that boundaries play. When someone crosses the line you set, you have every right to stand up for yourself and remind them of your limit, no matter who they are and no matter the perceived power dynamic.

Your boundaries will be different for different people in your life. A question your endocrinologist asks may not be appropriate for your mom to ask. Something you share with another person with T1D may not be relevant for you to talk about with your teacher.

You have to set boundaries with people in your life around T1D, including your health care team. When someone like a doctor crosses a boundary with you, sometimes the best option is to get the support you need by setting a very firm boundary and finding a new doctor.

Support from Others with T1D

Whenever I see a new patient, one of the first questions I always ask is whether they know any other people who have T1D. The vast majority tell me that I am one of the first people with T1D they have ever had a conversation with. Some say that they knew someone in high school or they have a distant cousin, but very few have a network of people with T1D they talk to regularly.

Connecting with other people with T1D can be a powerful experience. When you connect with other people with diabetes, you get to feel "normal" and to be around people who "get it." But the benefits of connection go far beyond having friends with T1D. There are many faces of support that go beyond being around other people like you. Maybe you don't need the "shoulder to cry on" type of support, and perhaps you don't want to spend time talking about diabetes. That's okay. The value of the diabetes community is multidimensional, including having your back in your time of need.

I want you to know there are other people out there who get you. I want you to know others experience the same highs, lows, frustration, and burnout as you do. These people know exactly how you feel and let you know they have your back with a simple smile or a nod.

You may be asking yourself: *Why would I want to connect with other people with T1D? I want my life to be less about diabetes, not more. If I'm part of the diabetes community, that means I'll have to spend more time talking about diabetes— and that's not what I want!*

Let me tell you a secret.

When people with T1D connect, there are times when diabetes is the focus. But most of the time, diabetes stays in the background. The mere fact that it's present is comforting. People with T1D are multidimensional, and being around others like them can let their personalities shine because diabetes is not at the forefront.

In addition to emotional support, others with T1D also can give you resources and information to make life with diabetes less stressful. Here are a few examples...

Supplies

You need a lot of supplies to manage T1D effectively. Sometimes you may run out of your diabetes supplies, the shipment may be delayed, or you lose your health insurance. If you don't have access to everything you need to manage your diabetes, things can quickly become stressful. Having a solid T1D support system can help. People with T1D tend to be generous with their resources and always willing to lend a hand when needed. Without connection to others with T1D, you're going to be on your own.

Recommendations

Need to find a doctor who will spend the time to listen to your concerns? A book to help change the way you think about T1D? A recipe for low-carb pancakes? The best way to find these resources is from other people with T1D. We all have found things that work for us, and we want to tell others about them. The only way we can share this information is when we have a connection with other T1Ds.

Tips and Tricks

Did you know you can extend your CGM sensor? Have you ever tried putting your pump site on your leg? Know that taking a brisk walk after a carb-heavy meal can help reduce your post-meal spike? The T1D community has millions of years of diabetes under its belt, and in that time, we've come up with some tricks to handle the curveballs diabetes throws us. Our collective knowledge is immense, and connecting with other people with T1D lets us spread the wealth.

Where to Find Support from Others With T1D

Here are some places where people with T1D can find support...

Social Media

The ability to connect in real time with others worldwide who also have T1D has been a game-changer. Need some insulin or diabetes supplies? Put a post on Facebook, and someone will offer to help within minutes. Need to vent? There are people out there who get it and will listen and empathize. Do you want to get your support as a passive observer, reading about other people's experiences so you don't feel so alone in yours? You can scroll to your heart's content.

Where to Find Support on Social Media

Facebook, Instagram, Twitter, and TikTok all have large communities of people with T1D. Search #T1D and #T1DLooksLikeMe to join the conversation.

DR. MARK'S T1D

I wasn't always active in the diabetes community. After I was diagnosed and people told me I should meet other people with T1D, several thoughts jumped to mind. I had this image of sitting around a table in a dingy, windowless room in the basement of some hospital where everyone would be comparing notes about their A1Cs, insulin-to-carb ratios, and correction factors. That sounded (and still sounds) awful to me. Second, if I wanted to find support from other T1Ds (and I did, even if I didn't want to admit it), I had no idea where to find it. Going to the type of support group I had conjured up in my mind was off the table, but I had nowhere else to turn.

Several years later, everything changed for me. I joined a kickboxing gym and started going to an early-morning class. And as I mentioned in the introduction of this book, one day after class, a woman about my age came up to me and said words that would change my life forever.

As I was stretching, she said, "You have type 1 diabetes!"

I looked up at her quizzically, wondering how she knew. Was it that obvious? She pointed to my pump site, visible as my shirt pulled up during my stretch. During this brief conversation, she mentioned she had a blog where she wrote about her life with T1D and encouraged me to check it out.

Over the next week, I devoured every single one of her blog posts. Then I went looking for more blogs to read. I didn't know it at the time, but that brief interaction with another person with T1D and the introduction to her blog was exactly what I needed— support in an unexpected way.

Reading her descriptions of her everyday experience of living with diabetes opened my eyes. I don't think I realized how alone I had been feeling. To have someone else describe what they were feeling and to be able to see my own experience mirrored there was powerful. I remember one blog where she described the small details of what *high blood sugar feels like. This feeling was one I had had numerous times but could never put into words. I could never describe to my wife what was happening to me. This post not only gave me evidence that I was not the only one who felt this way but also gave me the words I needed to share my experience with those closest to me.*

Simply put, meeting this woman at the gym, reading her blog, and then going down the rabbit hole of reading about other T1Ds was a catalyst that helped make diabetes easier to handle.

This experience taught me an important lesson I use every day in my work, even now as I am immersed in the T1D community. There are many faces of peer support for people with T1D, and there is no wrong way to get the help you need. You can do something as passive as picking up your phone and scrolling Instagram to being proactive and flying across the country for a weeklong conference—or anything in between.

Blogs and Podcasts

The support I got from reading that woman's blog was powerful and completely passive. I resonated with her experience simply by reading about it on my computer screen, and this made me feel heard and validated. After reading those posts, I knew I wasn't alone, and it pushed me to seek out more resources like it. Support doesn't need to be one-to-one, and sometimes it can be more effective when it is one-to-many. Passive support, like blogs and podcasts, provides the opportunity for people with T1D to feel validated and not so alone with a low barrier to entry. It also cracks the door for people looking for other forms of support.

Where to Find Blogs and Podcasts about T1D
Start by using your favorite search engine to find blogs and podcasts to give you the support you're looking for. And don't limit your search to the ones that have tens of thousands of readers or listeners. Maybe the content with the most significant impact for you will be the random thoughts about T1D someone wrote in the middle of the night and posted on their website. You also will come across T1D blogs and podcasts on social media, so be sure to keep an eye out there for content that speaks to you.

— — —

Looking for a podcast all about T1D & mental health?

Go to www.thediabetespsychologist.com/mypodcast or scan the code below to listen to The Diabetes Psychologist Podcast.

— — —

In-person Support

My mental image of in-person support has changed significantly over the years. It has gone from sitting around a poorly lit room in the basement of a hospital to hanging out in a bar or in the mountains with other people with T1D. Being around others with diabetes is a transformative experience. You're around other people who truly get you. Being around other T1Ds lets you get the support you need without having to ask. It just happens.

- - -

Looking for in-person support options?

Go to www.thediabetespsychologist.com/support or scan the code below for a list of resources.

- - -

──────── **CHAPTER 9 KEY TAKEAWAYS** ────────

- *Everyone with T1D needs support. Type 1 diabetes should never be a do-it-yourself condition.*

- *People with T1D need many types of support, including emotional, physical, logistical, and financial.*

- *Support can come from different groups of people, including friends and family, your health care team, and others with T1D.*

- *The only way to get the support you need with T1D is to ask for it.*

- *You need support from other people with T1D.*

- *Others with T1D can provide a type of support that people who don't have T1D can't. They can understand exactly what you're experiencing and how you feel.*

Chapter 10

YOU CAN HANDLE THE REALLY TOUGH STUFF

THE HUMAN CAPACITY FOR BURDEN IS LIKE BAMBOO—FAR MORE FLEXIBLE THAN YOU'D EVER BELIEVE AT FIRST GLANCE.

—JODI PICOULT

AFTER YOU IMPLEMENT all the skills you've learned in this book so far, there still may be times when T1D is tricky, and you find it difficult to handle.

If you follow the process I laid out in this book, T1D won't always be easy, but you'll be able to handle it. But if you're honest with yourself, there will be times when additional challenges come up, and you may start to think you can't handle them.

What do you do when T1D throws you a big curveball?

I can guarantee you there will be unexpected challenges with T1D in your future. And I am confident you can handle them, even when you have no idea what they look like and when they're going to happen.

I know you'll feel like you can't handle these situations. You're just getting steady on your feet with the day-to-day stress and annoyances of T1D. But what happens when something knocks you down, and you feel like you're right back where you started?

First, let's talk about what you can do to handle it when something knocks you to the ground. Then I'll give you some strategies to help you in specific situations.

When T1D throws something challenging your way, always go back to the basics. Recognize that you're in a tough spot. Don't try to sugarcoat it. Pretending like it doesn't suck does nothing to change the reality of the situation. To deal with this challenge, you need to face it head-on.

After acknowledging you're not in a great place, you can start handling it. If you need a refresher on the steps you can take to deal with the challenging emotions T1D throws your way, go back and re-read Chapter 7. You will find guidance that you can apply to even the most difficult situations with T1D.

There are many things that can happen to make T1D even more challenging than usual. Here are just a few of the challenges T1D may throw your way and some suggestions for what you can do to handle them when they do come up.

Diabetic Ketoacidosis

Diabetic ketoacidosis is a severe and often life-threatening complication from diabetes. When the body does not have enough insulin to break down glucose, it forces the body to start breaking down fat as fuel, releasing ketones into the body.

Symptoms of DKA include constant fatigue, nausea, vomiting, shortness of breath, fruity smell on the breath, flushed skin, and disorientation. DKA needs to be treated in the hospital. If you think there is any chance you are in DKA, seek medical attention immediately.

Going into DKA is the biggest nightmare of every person with T1D. You feel like death, and the only ticket to recovery is a stay in the ICU. After getting out of the hospital, you may have many feelings, including guilt, anxiety, and fear. You may be terrified of going into DKA again and feel like you're walking on eggshells around your diabetes.

How You Can Handle DKA

- **The past does not have to predict the future:** *After recovering from DKA, the scariest part is fear that it will happen again. You feel like a failure for going into DKA in the first place, and you may feel powerless to stop it from happening again. DKA is scary, but for most people, it's a rare occurrence. Just because you've been in DKA in the past doesn't mean it will happen again. Managing T1D is all about identifying patterns, and DKA doesn't have to be a pattern for you.*

- **Take simple steps to reduce your chance of going into DKA:** *You're not powerless to prevent DKA. You can take simple actions to significantly reduce the likelihood of going into DKA, including taking your insulin, monitoring your blood sugar, following your sick day plan, and checking for ketones. Work with your diabetes care team to* *figure out what these steps are for you. Keeping this in mind can help you deal with your anxiety that history will repeat itself and DKA will be a regular part of your life.*

Severe Lows

There is nothing like a severe low blood sugar to remind you how much T1D sucks. You start sweating through your clothes, feel weak in the knees, and the words coming out of your mouth stop making sense. The scariest part of a severe low is feeling out of control and worrying that you won't be able to take care of yourself and bring it back up.

How You Can Handle Your Anxiety about Lows

- **Accept the fact that you will go low:** *Blood sugar management is a balancing act, and if you take insulin, you most likely will go low every once in a while. This is normal. If you accept that you will go low from time to time, you can be ready to catch it and deal with it before you get into a dangerous situation.*

- **The past does not predict the future:** *Like with DKA, a severe low in the past does not mean it has to happen again. Our brains are wired to focus on the scary things and forget about most times when nothing happens. When anxiety about having a severe low takes over your mind, take a step back and remember the times when nothing bad happened—and trust me, there are a lot of those times.*

- **Trust your body:** *Your low symptoms are not pleasant. And this is a good thing. These symptoms let you know something is going on that you need to pay attention to. When you trust your body, you can see that you can deal with lows when you have them.*

- **Trust your technology:** *Diabetes technology has come a long way in recent years, and now many people have access to tools that can help keep their blood sugars even more stable. Continuous glucose monitors give you information about your current blood sugar, as well as where your blood sugar is going and how quickly it's moving. Trusting your CGM to do its job helps you handle your anxiety around having a bad low.*

- **Trust yourself:** *If you do go low, trust that you can take care of yourself. Trust that you'll be able to recognize when your blood sugar is low—either on your own or with the help of technology—and when this happens, that you'll be capable of treating it. Lows are scary. However, your fear doesn't have to rob you of your ability to stop what you're doing and have some glucose to bring your blood sugar back into range. You've done it many times before, and you can use your past successes to help you trust that you'll be able to take care of your lows when they happen again.*

Difficulty Sleeping

Restful sleep with T1D can be hard to come by. You wake

up when your blood sugar is high. You wake up when your blood sugar is low. You may have trouble falling asleep because you are worried about high or low blood sugar in the middle of the night. And let's not even talk about the alerts and alarms that wake you up.

When you don't sleep well, your blood sugars, mood, and energy level suffer. You want to figure out what to do, but nothing you do seems to work.

How You Can Handle Sleep Problems

- **Manage your blood sugar:** *If your blood sugars are all over the place, sleep will be challenging. You don't feel well, and your blood sugars keep your mind active, making sleep elusive. The first step to better sleep with T1D is working to keep your blood sugars in range. Leaning into your diabetes management reduces the chance wacky blood sugars will get in the way of your sleep and increases your confidence you will be safe going to sleep.*

- **Know your anxiety about sleep with T1D is not unfounded:** *You're not crazy for being anxious about sleeping with T1D. It is perfectly reasonable to be nervous. Instead of letting it paralyze you, try using this anxiety to help set yourself up for success.*

- **Make small changes:** *Even small changes can make a big difference in your sleep with T1D. For example, try cutting out your late-night snack so*

*you can go to bed with your blood sugar close to
your target. Go to sleep with little to no insulin
on board, use the technology you have access to,
and make sure you have glucose close to your bed.
With some planning, you can take simple steps to
keep yourself safe.*

- **Get out of bed:** *If you're having trouble sleeping, get out of bed. Anxiety leads to sleep problems, and sometimes your actions keep them
going. When you're in bed and can't fall asleep,
your mind starts to associate lying in bed with
being awake. Anytime you get in bed, you think
you should be awake. The best way to break
this association and reprogram your mind is to
get out of bed if you can't fall asleep after about
fifteen minutes. Do something tedious and then
go back to bed and try again when you start
getting sleepy.*

- **Practice self-compassion:** *Sleep with T1D can
be tricky. Just because something is hard doesn't
make it impossible. If you have a difficult time
sleeping because of diabetes, try not to be too hard
on yourself. The more compassionate you can be
with yourself, the easier it will be to fall asleep and
stay asleep, even if your CGM starts beeping in the
middle of the night.*

Complications

Type 1 diabetes can get complicated in more ways than one.
You hear about what can happen if you don't manage your

blood sugar, and you know that diabetes-related complications can occur even when you keep your blood sugars in a
good range. If you haven't developed complications, you may
be anxious about what might happen to you in the future.

I sincerely hope you never have to deal with diabetes complications, and if you have already developed complications,
I hope they don't get worse. Nonetheless, thinking about
and dealing with diabetes-related complications can be
hard to handle.

How You Can Handle Complications

- **Get support:** *You should not have to deal with
  T1D alone, and you absolutely should not deal
  with complications alone. There is so much that
  goes into having T1D-related complications, both
  emotionally and physically. You need support from
  people who care about you to help you handle
  living with complications. Hopefully, you can get
  the support you need from your close friends and
  family, others dealing with T1D-related complications, and your health care team.*

- **Know you're not alone:** *If you do develop a
  complication, you're not alone. Many other people
  live with complications and have felt the same way
  you're feeling right now. Knowing you're not alone
  in your experience makes it easier to deal with the
  fact that complications suck.*

- **Allow yourself to mourn:** *Getting diagnosed with
  a complication is hard news to swallow. Handling*

this news and what comes next can take time. You may feel all kinds of emotions; whatever you're feeling is normal. Give yourself permission to be upset and mourn the loss in this diagnosis. An essential part of handling T1D-related complications is to acknowledge that T1D sucks.

- **Don't let your stories run away:** *Diabetes complications suck. They also add fuel to the stories you tell yourself about what T1D means about you. These stories often include subplots of shame, blame, and regret. Of course, complications are never your desired outcome. However, you also want to make sure you don't put more meaning on developing a complication than it deserves. If you notice your stories make your complications more challenging to deal with, bring your mind back to the present moment. Don't let complications suck any more than they already do.*

- **Don't give up:** *If you develop diabetes-related complications, you may feel like giving up on your diabetes management. Whatever you do, don't throw in the towel. There are still things you can do to manage complications and prevent them from getting worse. Your behavior still matters.*

Sexual Dysfunction

Sexual problems caused by diabetes are one of the complications we don't talk about enough. Experiencing diabetes-related sexual dysfunction can be embarrassing, or worse, devastating. But as you know, just because it sucks doesn't mean you can't handle it.

How You Can Handle Sexual Dysfunction

- **Call it what it is:** *There is no way to sugarcoat sexual problems caused by T1D. To handle it, you have to accept what's going on and its impact on you and your relationship(s). After you call it for what it is and recognize it sucks, you'll be in a place to change what you can and accept that which you cannot change.*

- **Seek medical treatment:** *When you have a realistic idea about what's going on and what you can do about it, there's more hope you can handle it. Some treatments have the potential to help you regain sexual functioning. Talk to your doctor about what options are available to you.*

- **Know you're not alone:** *It can be lonely to deal with sexual dysfunction. You may feel like you're the only person dealing with this challenge. You're not alone; many other people are in the same situation and understand how you feel. This solidarity can make this big challenge easier to handle.*

Difficult Health Care Providers

Your diabetes care team plays a significant role in helping you manage T1D, but a lot of times, they never talk about the stress of living with the condition. Sometimes, they may even say things that make the emotional burden of T1D even worse. Unfortunately, comments about how you're not trying hard enough to manage your diabetes, using scare tactics to push you toward taking care of yourself, or even scolding you for high numbers are not uncommon stories.

A poor relationship with your endocrinologist can lead to feelings of guilt and shame, making it more challenging to handle T1D.

How You Can Handle a Difficult Provider

- **Make your needs known:** *Don't be scared to let your health care team know what you need from them. Your providers may be so focused on your blood sugars that they ignore your emotional health, which, of course, affects your blood sugars. They may need you to guide them and tell them what they can do to help you.*

- **Give constructive feedback:** *If your diabetes care team says things that aren't helpful or worse, that make you feel bad about yourself, don't be scared to let them know. They may have no idea how they come across, and your feedback can help them adjust their style and empower you to stand up for yourself. Keep in mind that health care providers are human and make mistakes sometimes. Constructive feedback is always appropriate because it helps them learn how to provide the best support possible to people with T1D.*

- **Find a new health care provider:** *Remember who the most important member of your health care team is.* **Hint:** *It's you! Your diabetes care team is there to coach and guide you on how to dial in your blood sugars. They are not in charge of you. Guilt and shame have no place in your diabetes care. You are the captain of your diabe-*

tes care team, and you get to call the shots. Never forget, if your diabetes care team is not giving you the support you need, this may be a sign it's time to find a new team.

Finances

Diabetes is expensive, and the cost of managing T1D only adds to your stress. If you're worried about how to pay for the supplies that keep you alive, you're going to have a hard time handling it.

How You Can Handle the Financial Stress

- **Lean into the diabetes community:** *I do not know many people in the diabetes community who would not help another T1D in need. Connecting with other T1Ds can make you feel more secure and, hopefully, put you in a position where you will never have to worry about going without the supplies you need to stay alive and healthy.*

- **Tell your health care team:** *There is no shame in admitting you struggle to afford your insulin or other supplies needed to manage diabetes. Your diabetes care team and your primary care provider may have samples, discount cards, and other programs and resources you can use to help you pay for your supplies. However, they cannot help you if they don't know you're struggling.*

- **Breathe:** *The financial aspect of T1D is stressful. Staying calm will help you navigate these issues with a clear head. If you feel overwhelmed paying* *for the tools you need to stay alive, take a deep breath. Of course, a deep breath will not put any money in your bank account, but taking a break can help you deal with these challenges as effectively as possible.*

- **Find your voice:** *The only way living with T1D is going to become more affordable is if you make your voice heard. Small actions can have a significant impact. Sign a petition, post about it on social media, talk to your friends, family, and elected leaders about this issue. Your voice matters, and using your voice can help you handle the stress.*

Insurance

If you live in the United States, insurance is likely the bane of your existence—hours on the phone, only to be told you're not talking to the correct department, and appeal after appeal to get them to pay for the brand of insulin that works for you. In theory, your insurance company is there to help reduce the financial burden of T1D, but there is a cost that includes your time, patience, and sanity. To put it nicely, your health insurance company makes life with diabetes a lot more complicated than it needs to be.

How You Can Handle Insurance Stress

- **Find a doctor who will help**: *When dealing with insurance, you need someone who will go to bat for you to get the tools you need covered. Once you find a doctor who will make phone calls, file appeals, and do everything necessary to help you, don't ever let them go.*

- **Use available resources:** *Insurance companies have care navigators who can help you get the resources you need. Use them. Call your insurance company for information on the resources they offer.*

- **Be the squeaky wheel:** *In my experience, if you make enough noise, insurance companies will give you what you need to manage your diabetes. Don't be afraid to ask. And if the answer is no, ask again. Sometimes the only way to get what you need is to request it.*

- **Learn from others' experiences:** *Unfortunately, many of us have dealt with insurance companies, and some folks have had success. Connect with others to find out what they did to help them win their battles, big and small, with insurance companies.*

——— CHAPTER 10 KEY TAKEAWAYS ———

- *Even with the best coping skills, T1D will still throw you curveballs. These may include:*

  - *DKA*

  - *Severe lows*

  - *Sleep challenges*

  - *Complications*

  - *Sexual dysfunction*

  - *Unsupportive health care providers*

- *Finances*

- *Insurance*

- *It may not feel like it, but you have the tools you need to handle the toughest of these challenges.*

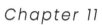

Chapter 11

WHEN YOU NEED PROFESSIONAL HELP

ASK FOR HELP. NOT BECAUSE YOU ARE WEAK. BUT BECAUSE YOU WANT TO REMAIN STRONG.

—LES BROWN

THERE MAY BE times when you should not handle the stress of T1D on your own.

I hope this book has given you the tools to handle many of the challenges diabetes throws your way. But there may be times when you need support from a mental health professional.

How to Figure Out if You Need Therapy

If you have diabetes and you're struggling, how do you know if you should get professional help?

The answer to this question is not always cut and dried, but here are a few questions you can ask yourself that may help you figure it out.

Is your stress impacting your ability to manage diabetes?
One of the most common reasons people seek professional help is because they're feeling frustrated and defeated by diabetes. These feelings make it hard for them to get motivated to check their blood sugar and take insulin. If the feeling of being overwhelmed impacts your ability to manage your blood sugars, you might benefit from professional support.

Are your struggles with T1D hurting your relationships?
For example, do other people tell you they're worried about you or don't want to be around you because you're moody, irritable, or just not yourself? This feedback may be a sign you could benefit from professional help.

Is the stress of diabetes making it difficult to do things that are important to you?
Mental health treatment might be helpful if T1D is getting in the way of living your life and stopping you from doing the things you want to do, especially if you still feel stuck after trying to move forward on your own.

Have you tried the strategies covered in this book or other things that could help, and they still don't seem to be working?
This book has tools that I know will help you. I also know these tools may not be enough and that you may need more help. If you have tried these and other strategies and you're still struggling, it doesn't mean things won't improve. It may be a signal you need a different kind of support.

Do you have non-diabetes-related mental health challenges that exacerbate the stress of T1D or make it harder to manage T1D?

Emotional challenges occur for all kinds of reasons. Diabetes is one, but it's certainly not the only one. Family issues, relationship problems, or past trauma are just some reasons why your emotional health is not in a great place right now. No matter where these challenges come from, they impact you and probably affect your ability to manage your diabetes. They probably also make any challenges you're experiencing with diabetes more difficult to handle.

If you answered yes to any of the questions above, you might benefit from talking to a mental health professional.

There is never any harm in making an appointment with a mental health professional to find out more about therapy and whether it could help you. With any kind of mental health treatment, you are always in the driver's seat. Making an appointment doesn't commit you to long-term therapy. It's just a way for you to get the information you need to decide whether professional support could help you.

You may benefit from professional help, but for most people, it's not the only option. This book lays out the types of things you can try on your own. If you feel you need therapy, I highly recommend you seek it out. However, I also want to make sure you have the tools you need to think beyond therapy.

You Need a Therapist Who Understands T1D
Not all therapy is created equal for people with T1D. If what you're struggling with is diabetes-related, you need a therapist who understands T1D.

If T1D is the reason you're seeking therapy, a therapist who doesn't know much about diabetes may have a hard time understanding this issue, and many may not know how to help. If a provider is going to treat things like diabetes burnout, fear of hypoglycemia, and diabulimia, they need to have an in-depth understanding of diabetes to be helpful. Without knowing anything about T1D, they probably won't know what questions to ask or where to start.

Finding a Therapist Who Understands T1D

If you're looking for a therapist specializing in diabetes, the best place to start is with your endocrinologist or diabetes educator. A lot of times, they can refer you to a therapist who specializes in this. You also can do a Google search or ask other people with diabetes for a recommendation. Unfortunately, there aren't enough of us out there, so if you find someone who has helped you, let your doctor and others know about this therapist.

Another helpful resource is the American Diabetes Association (ADA). They developed a mental health provider training program and created a directory of providers who understand the mental health challenges of living with type 1 diabetes. **You can find the ADA Mental Health Provider Directory at: https://professional.diabetes.org/mhp_listing**

What Therapy Is Like

A lot of people wonder what happens in therapy. Therapy isn't a magic bullet; it's hard work. But it can be a safe, supportive place to work on whatever challenges you face. A therapist will try to help you develop the skills to better tolerate the challenges of living with diabetes, problem-solve complex issues, and understand how your thoughts affect your emotions and behavior.

When to Consider Medication

There may come a time when medication would be helpful as you work to handle the stress of T1D. It also is possible you will never need medication or you may benefit from taking medication right now. I want to make sure you have the information you need about medicine if you ever are at an emotional point where you need it.

Whenever I suggest medication to my patients, I almost always get some degree of pushback. I get it. Thinking about taking medication that affects your brain is scary, especially when you already are feeling overwhelmed. People tell me they think they should be able to deal with the pressure on their own, and they see medication as a quick Band-Aid and not a long-term solution.

Here is how I describe medication…

Medication is not going to make your stress, anxiety, or burnout go away. But what it can do is get you to a place where you can handle these feelings more effectively. I compare experiencing these challenging emotions to walking through a field filled with grass taller than your head. You have no idea where you're going and no way to figure out how to get to a better place. But if you had a step stool, you would be able to peek over the top of the grass and get an idea of where you need to go. The step stool puts you in a place where you can chart a path forward. Medication is like a step stool. It doesn't make your challenges with T1D go away, but it can put you in a place where you can better help yourself.

I have seen how much these medications have helped people get to a place where they can better handle T1D. In the end, the decision is yours. You always have the final say whether you want to take these types of medications. I just want to make sure you know this is an available tool if you choose to use it.

The Bottom Line

Living with T1D is tough. If you're having a hard time handling T1D on your own, you're not alone. This is nothing to be ashamed of or embarrassed about. There is specialized mental health treatment available for people with T1D. If you feel like you can't deal with the stress of T1D on your own and would benefit from professional help, take advantage of it.

Recognizing when you're having trouble handling T1D on your own is a sign that you can handle it; you just may need a little help.

If you are in crisis and need help immediately, call the National Suicide Prevention Lifeline at 800-273-8255.

─────── **CHAPTER 11 KEY TAKEAWAYS** ───────

- *There may be times when you can't handle T1D on your own, and you need professional help.*

- *Seeking help when you need it is a sign of strength.*

- *Therapy is appropriate if T1D impacts your ability to function at the level you desire. For example, if your T1D-related stress affects your ability to work, your relationships, or your diabetes management, therapy can help.*

- *If you seek therapy for a concern related to T1D, it's critical to find a therapist who understands T1D.*

- *Medication doesn't make your problems go away, but it may help you see a path forward if you're struggling.*

Chapter 12

BEYOND HANDLING T1D

*YOU AIN'T SEEN NOTHING YET, AND
THE BEST IS YET TO COME.*

—*MICHAEL JACKSON*

WHEN YOU CAN handle type 1 diabetes, the stress of T1D is no longer a barrier in your life. Instead, it becomes your companion. It's with you, but it's not bothering you. You can coexist peacefully with your diabetes.

Of course, there will be times when diabetes doesn't bother you and times when it is more stressful. And now you have the tools to carry the burden of T1D with you and not let it get in your way, no matter what season you find yourself in.

The skills and tools in this book are all about creating systems and processes to deal with all the challenges that diabetes throws at you. These skills are essential for your emotional health with T1D because they give you the freedom and flexibility that you want in your life. Simply put, these tools and skills help you react to diabetes more effectively.

If you can react to the pressure of T1D even just a little better than you could before, you have made significant progress. Keep up the good work!

People sometimes ask, is handling the stress of T1D enough, or can you aim for more? And if the answer to the latter question is yes, then what's the next step?

Diabetes is a condition that requires management. You manage your blood sugars and your emotions. You may even have to manage your health care team. Management is all about working within the current system in the most effective way possible. And right now, your system includes a dysfunctional pancreas, which leads to frustration and stress. And, unfortunately, this system shows no sign of going away anytime soon.

But what if you could manage diabetes and your emotions but also do more? The barriers that once got in your way are now gone. Now that you're feeling more freedom and flexibility in your life, what if you could get out of the box of your current life and prepare for a future you couldn't previously have imagined? Your next step is to think about what's possible in your life.

You can move beyond a mindset of management and into a place of possibility. You are in charge of your life, and nobody but you gets to decide where you go and what you do.

Why are you ready to take on this leadership role in your life right now? Because now you are honest with yourself that T1D sucks and confident that you can handle it!

YOUR NEXT STEPS

CONGRATULATIONS! YOU NOW have a solid foundation to handle any stress T1D throws your way.

You are off to a great start!

Where do you go from here? How do you continue to practice and refine the skills you've learned to manage the emotional burden of T1D?

I wrote this book to give you all the information and tools you need to handle the stress of T1D. However, knowledge and tools are necessary but not sufficient for handling T1D. To deal with the challenges of diabetes effectively, you have to implement the skills I introduced in this book.

Your immediate next step is to take what you've learned and put it into action—today! Start implementing your new tools in your way so you can find the freedom and flexibility you are looking for.

If you need a refresher on what you learned, I encourage you to go back and re-read sections of this book. I wrote this book to be a reference that you can go back and review anytime.

As you start putting your new skills and tools into action, you may find you need some additional support and concrete next steps. If that's the case for you, I have you covered.

Here are some options to help you decide what specific next step is right for you:

Option #1: Track your progress
You probably have already made more progress than you think. Monitoring your progress is a great way to stay on track implementing your new tools in your life with T1D because you can see the impact of your behavior. If you find that you're not making the progress you want, it may be a sign you need additional support.

Go to www.thediabetespsychologist.com/progress or scan the code below to download your T1D & Mental Health progress tracker!

Option #2: Join *The Diabetes Psychologist Membership*
Would you benefit from ongoing support to help you navigate the stress of living with T1D? The Diabetes Psychologist

Membership gives you the tools, resources, and skills you need to deal effectively with all the stress T1D throws your way. In this monthly membership, you will get the support, accountability, resources, and community you need to navigate the stress of living with type 1 diabetes.

Go to www.thediabetespsycholgoist.com/membership or scan the code below to join The Diabetes Psychologist Membership!

Option #3: Enroll in *Get Unstuck with T1D*

Do you want to take what you've learned in this book and dive deeper? Are you looking for a guided process to help you implement the skills you learned in this book? *Get Unstuck* with T1D is a 6-week digital program that will take you through a step-by-step process to put your skills into action. This program includes videos, presentations, worksheets, and resources to give you everything you need to make the transformation you are looking for.

Go to www.thediabetespsychologist.com/getunstuck or scan the code on the next page to enroll in Get Unstuck with T1D!

No matter what you decide your next step is, take action! Invest the time and effort in yourself to see what's possible in your life with T1D.

Because even though diabetes sucks, you **can** handle it!

GLOSSARY

A1C	A blood test that tells you your average blood sugar level over the past three months. The result is reported as a percentage, and most people with T1D have an A1C goal of below 7%. This test can also be referred to as hemoglobin A1c and HbA1c.
Basal insulin (also called long-acting insulin)	Insulin that works in the background to keep blood sugars stable throughout the day. The most common basal insulin brands are Basaglar, Lantus, Levemir, Toujeo, and Tresiba.
Basal rate	The rate an insulin pump gives small doses of short-acting insulin throughout the day to keep blood sugars stable.
Blood glucose level	The amount of sugar (glucose) in the blood. Elevated blood glucose levels indicate a person has diabetes. A typical blood glucose range for people who do not have diabetes is 70mg/dL–140mg/dL. American Diabetes Association guidelines suggest people with diabetes try to keep their blood glucose level between 70mg/dL–180mg/dL.
Blood glucose meter	A small device that measures how much glucose is in the blood. It works by placing a small drop of blood from the finger on a test strip.

Bolus	A dose of insulin taken before eating or to bring down a high blood sugar. A bolus can be given as an injection or with an insulin pump.
Certified Diabetes Care and Education Specialist (CDCES)	A healthcare professional trained to educate people with diabetes about diabetes management, medication, and diet. You may also hear them referred to as Certified Diabetes Educators (CDE).
Continuous glucose monitor (CGM)	A device that continuously tracks blood glucose levels using a sensor worn on the body. A transmitter wirelessly sends the blood glucose data to a monitor, where you can look at it anytime. The most common CGM brands are Abbott, Dexcom, and Medtronic.
Diabetic ketoacidosis (DKA)	A severe and often life-threatening complication from diabetes. When the body does not have enough insulin to break down glucose, it forces the body to start breaking down fat as fuel, releasing ketones into the body.
Endocrinologist	A doctor who specializes in treating people with diabetes.
Glucose	A simple sugar the body breaks down from food and uses as the primary fuel for the body's cells.
Infusion set	Thin plastic tubing that connects an insulin pump to the body. At the end of the tubing, a soft, flexible cannula or a stainless-steel needle attaches to the body and delivers insulin.

Insulin	A hormone made by the pancreas that allows glucose to enter cells and produce energy.
Insulin-to-carb ratio	The number of units of insulin one needs to take when eating a specific number of grams of carbohydrates.
Insulin pump	A small, battery-powered device that automatically delivers small doses of rapid-acting insulin continuously (basal rate) and larger amounts of rapid-acting when food is eaten or to correct high blood sugar (bolus). The most common insulin pump brands are Medtronic, Omnipod, and Tandem Diabetes Care.
High blood sugar	A condition that occurs when there is excess glucose in the blood. Most people who do not have diabetes never have a blood sugar over 140mg/dl. If you have diabetes, talk to your doctor about what a high blood sugar level is for you. Blood sugar levels can be high with or without symptoms. Common symptoms of high blood sugar include fatigue, dry mouth, feeling heavy or slow, excess thirst, frequent urination, and blurred vision. High blood sugar occurs when there is not enough insulin to deal with the glucose in the body. Many factors raise blood sugar levels, including food, stress, and hormones. For people with type 1 diabetes, high blood sugar is treated by taking insulin.

Low blood sugar	Sometimes referred to as hypoglycemia. A condition that occurs when one's blood sugar is lower than 70 mg/dL. Causes of low blood sugar include taking too much insulin, not eating enough carbohydrates, and physical activity. Symptoms of low blood sugar include hunger, nervousness, shakiness, perspiration, dizziness or light-headedness, sleepiness, and confusion. If left untreated, hypoglycemia may lead to unconsciousness. Low blood sugar is treated by consuming simple carbohydrates such as glucose tablets or juice. It can also be treated with glucagon if the person is unconscious or unable to swallow.
Mealtime insulin	See rapid-acting insulin.
Multiple daily injections (MDI)	A method of treating diabetes where one injects both long-acting insulin (usually once per day) and rapid-acting insulin (multiple times per day for food and to correct high blood sugar).
Pump site	The place where an insulin pump attaches to the body on the skin.

Rapid-acting insulin	The type of insulin taken before meals and to correct high blood sugars. Rapid-acting insulin starts to bring down blood sugar about 15 minutes after it is administered, peaks within one to two hours, and continues working for two to four hours. Common brands of rapid-acting insulin include Admelog, Afrezza (inhaled), Apidra, Fiasp, Humalog, Lyumjev, and Novolog.
Type 1 diabetes (T1D)	A chronic auto-immune condition in which the pancreas does not produce insulin.